"Pink Hell"

Breast Cancer Sucks

Dr. Melissa Bailey

Published by Richter Publishing LLC www.richterpublishing.com

Editors: Casey Cavanagh, Nora Sarsour, Monica San Nicolas & Mandi Weems

ISBN: 0692533680
ISBN-13: 9780692533680

PINK HELL

DISCLAIMER

This book is designed to provide information on dealing with breast cancer only. This information is provided and sold with the knowledge that the publisher and author do not offer any legal or medical advice. In the case of a need for any such expertise, consult with the appropriate professional. This book does not contain all information available on the subject. This book has not been created to be specific to any individual's or organization's situation or needs. Every effort has been made to make this book as accurate as possible. However, there may be typographical and/ or content errors. Therefore, this book should serve only as a general guide and not as the ultimate source of subject information. This book contains information that might be dated and is intended only to educate and entertain. The author and publisher shall have no liability or responsibility to any person or entity regarding any loss or damage incurred, or alleged to have incurred, directly or indirectly, by the information contained in this book. You hereby agree to be bound by this disclaimer or you may return this book within the guarantee time period for a full refund. In the interest of full disclosure, this book contains affiliate links that might pay the author or publisher a commission upon any purchase from the company. While the author and publisher take no responsibility for the business practices of these companies and or the performance of any product or service, the author or publisher has used the product or service and makes a recommendation in good faith based on that experience. All characters appearing in this work are fictitious. Any resemblance to real persons, living or dead, is purely coincidental.

DEDICATION

This book is dedicated to my parents,
Ed and Louanne Bailey.
Because of the solid foundation of unconditional love you have provided
me, I have been able to succeed without fear of failure knowing that
you are always there to pick me up should I fall.

CONTENTS

INTRODUCTION

This is a journal of my adventures through breast cancer. Even though I'm a licensed clinical psychologist and work within the medical community, I had no idea that my going through cancer would have such an impact on my life and family. It's one of those things that you think will never happen to you. You feel sad for other people's stories, but never truly stop and think how it would affect *you*.

Within these pages, I document everything that happened in my life—from the moment I was diagnosed until I knew I was going to survive. Cancer wasn't going to get the best of me. Struggling through the pink hell of it all, I was going to come out on the other end.

I hope these stories help many other women who are dealing with their own illness. It's not an easy voyage, but if we can laugh along the way, it makes the pain a little bit easier to tolerate.

Sincerely,

Dr. Melissa Bailey

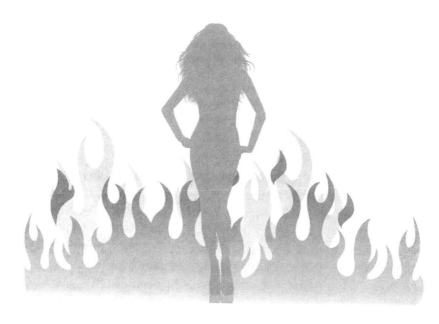

1 THE BEGINNING

April — May 4, 2010

I'm going to be 40 this year, and I'm not thrilled about it. A thought recently crossed my mind that I probably should go to a doctor because I'm pretty sure that a lot of "old people" check-up type stuff starts at age 40. I rarely go to the doctor. Actually, I work with doctors. I'm a licensed clinical psychologist, and I help consult people for weight loss surgery and other medical procedures, such as organ transplants. I'm constantly either chatting with physicians, in the hospital environment, or dealing with the patients. During my time off, the last place I want to be is in a medical environment. I want to be with my family relaxing. I figure if I'm around the hospital enough, the benefits will just rub off on me, right? Isn't that enough?

The last time I went to the doctor for personal reasons was when I had my daughter—5 years ago. I'm healthy except for allergies. But a little voice inside me tells me that I should really find a primary care doctor. After all, I recently I felt a lump in my left breast. I didn't think too much about it because, well, I have lumpy breasts. Apparently a lifetime on birth control pills can do that.

Reluctantly, I went to meet with my new doctor, Dr. Primary Care A lovely woman, probably about my mother's age. She did the usual medical history and such. I mentioned the lump. She said to come back for a "well woman check" and that she would order all of the appropriate womanly tests.

In the meantime, she had normal blood panels drawn on me. The blood tests reported that I'm completely healthy. No problems with high blood pressure, high cholesterol, nothing. Except that I have a severe vitamin D deficiency.

Two weeks later, on Wednesday, April 28th, I have the well-woman check with Dr. PCP. It reminds me of the story my dad tells before he goes to his urologist. Basically, they make the customary small talk for a while until the doctor "gets that look on his face," upon which my dad knows it's time to drop the pants. Of course, you have to hear my dad tell it with his sound effects and that Southern drawl of his.

Thinking of my father makes me giggle to myself as I sit and wait for the test to ensue. Her cold hands touch my flesh, and she also feels the lump in my left breast. She says I need to get a mammogram and an ultrasound. The laughter and my father fade with the seriousness of what may be more than just adverse effects to long-term birth control consumption.

Emotionless, my doctor tells me I have to go downtown because they have the "special" equipment. Great, I figure, how much more time out of my life am I going to have to spend on this? So, I call the imaging place immediately to get this over with and mention that my doctor referred me to them because I have a lump. Surprisingly, the woman on the other end of the phone says that she just happens to have a 12:30pm appointment for me today. What? Who has same-day appointments? I can't get my dry cleaning done the same day, but I can have my breasts smashed into small pancakes in about an hour.

Seeing that this is my first mammogram, I really didn't know what to expect. I enter the "Women's Center" area of the building, and everything is dripping pink. Pink walls, pink ribbons, even the employees are in pink scrubs. It was like a cupcake exploded in this place. I sign in and hardly have a chance to peruse the magazines when my name is called up for registration. The woman (wearing pink) behind the counter asks if this is my first mammogram. I tell her it is, and then she says how she *would* tell me that it's really easy. But the last time she told that to someone, they had a horrible time.

After registering, I was led into a back waiting area. I felt like I was entering some sort of private club. I was handed a spa-type gown and told to change, put my gown on, and wait in a different waiting room.

This waiting room had free bottled water and updated magazines. I then stripped down to everything but my underwear and put my clothes and purse in the little locker I was given. I went to sit in the private club waiting room and soon realized that everyone else in the room had on their shorts and high heel sandals on. Damn, now I'm sitting here almost totally naked and chilly so I went back to the locker, with my key hanging off the pink key chain, to get my shorts and shoes and put them back on.

My name finally is called by a nice woman who looks like she could have been my high school algebra teacher. Again, the small talk starts. "Is this your first mammogram?" and "Isn't the weather nice today?" She pretty much says anything to get my mind off what's she's about to do to my nice, soft bosoms. Once we get into the mammogram room there is a huge, tall machine with crystal plates on it. This is where the pancaking begins. Here comes the second set of hands on my breasts today. The tech starts putting stickers on my nipples. They really should have a pamphlet in the waiting room that cautions: *Expect to be fondled at least a dozen times during your visit today, and don't mind our happy stickers that will tear your nipples off after the procedure!*

The tech grabs my breast and puts it between plates, literally smashing it into a form I had no idea was possible. I joke with her that she must have punctured a couple of implants this way. With complete flat affect, she says, "No, not yet." Tough crowd. After she is done stretching out my breasts so they seem like they are hanging lower than when I came in, she says that she is going to ask the radiologist if she wants another view before I get my ultrasound.

I ask, "Why, see anything interesting?"

No response.

Do all the techs get schooled playing Texas Hold 'em? Because they have the best poker faces I've ever seen. She leaves, and then comes back. "No, doctor is fine with the films."

Next, I'm led to a room where another technician gets to fondle my breasts, but this time with warm K-Y jelly. She is a small, Asian woman who has a thick accent. I ask her if she has been doing this long. She basically tells me she has been doing it a long time and not to worry.

She then tells me that even after she finishes the ultrasound that usually the doctor wants to come in and do an ultrasound herself. I ask, "Is that because she doesn't like you?" She responded with a sly smile, "No, everyone likes me." A woman after my own heart.

Poker face Dr. Radiologist comes in and gets to play with my greased up breasts soon after. In the tone from the teacher of *Ferris Buller's Day Off*, she says, "You need to have a biopsy tomorrow."

The next day?! Why so soon? What's the emergency? What did they see on those scans? Everything that can race through my mind does, yet no one will tell me anything.

At this point, I'm introduced to the "Patient Navigator", who starts to tell me all about the biopsy and that she has to get a referral from my primary care physician and authorization from the insurance company. She floats out the door, leaving me to myself in a nice La-Z-Boy chair, where I can sit and think about what this all means. As I recline in my confusion, she returns to proclaim that she got the authorization, but can't get me in until Friday. Then she calmly asks, "Do you have any questions?"

Of course I do. Do I have cancer?

But no one wants to address that with me. No one wants to set my mind at ease. At this point, the thoughts are racing quicker than my heartbeats. As I leave the building, I call my mother, and she reassures me not to worry. Apparently 80 percent of breast lumps are non-cancerous. Both she and my grandmother have had benign cysts. Aren't I lucky that I won that genetic lottery? Next, I call my doctor's office just to get a confirmation on what is happening. The medical assistant tells me the same stat, 80 percent of lumps are benign. I respond that I couldn't get them to crack a smile, let alone give me any statistics.

Without any real answers, the waiting game begins.

Friday comes around and I'm really not that concerned. I have patients to call and reports to write. Again I come to the imaging center, and they are freakishly nice. However, I'm a tad bit paranoid; they must know something I don't. I'm brought back to change, but this time I feel like an old pro. I don't completely undress and go topless with the spa robe. An extremely cheerful ultrasound tech brings me back so she can again K-Y me up. She goes through the whole consenting process with me in regard to the biopsy. I'm not really sure what she said. My mind was not really functioning at that point, but I did notice the big ass needle they were going to use. I guess my fixation on it gave my worries away. "Oh, the casing makes it seem much bigger than it is," said the tech. Easy for her to say.

Dr. Poker Face comes in to start the procedure. She again asks me if I have any questions. I was not sure if at that point I was supposed to have questions. I did ask how long it would take to get back the report. "By Tuesday or Wednesday at the latest. We send the final report to your primary care doctor."

So, in other words, she was saying: "Don't ask us anything."

More waiting. I have to say that I really didn't think much about the biopsy, really assuming that it was just going to be a cyst. After all, that is what my mom said, and doesn't mother know best? I again called the medical assistant at my doctor's office to tell her to look for the report and let her know what number she can call me at when she gets it. Over the weekend, my daughter had some weird skin infection, so I was more focused on that. I had to cancel the first day of my business trip to take her to the pediatrician.

The following day, I have the phone strapped to my hip. I decide to go on my business trip and just fly in for the day to do some assessments. About an hour after I land and get my rental car, my phone rings with my doctor's office number on the screen. I pick it up and damn, it's not the medical assistant. It's the doctor. Never a good sign. "Oh, I'm so sorry. I just saw this report. Do you want to come in and talk about it?"

Talk about it? Talk about what? No one has said anything to me, even though I've been the one getting molested, poked, and prodded. I tell her that I have no idea what it says. She seems shocked that the imaging center didn't tell me. Apparently it's the pretty-in-pink girls, the cupcake explosion center, who are supposed to give you the life-or-death sentence.

She slowly tells me that it's cancer, breast cancer, metaplastic breast cancer, and she is not even sure what type it is because she hasn't seen this kind before.

I stop hearing her voice on the other end of the phone. I sink into what seems to be a dark tunnel where I'm alone, and everything starts going in slow motion. Time almost stops. My brain is trying to comprehend the words that are coming out of her mouth.

Not only do I have cancer, but I have some crazy type that is rare?

My heart drops into my stomach, and it twists with confusion and fear. I feel like I'm going to be sick. I can only mutter a few words back to the doctor, mentioning that I'm out of town but will manage to be at her office in the afternoon.

Panic sets in, and I start to call everyone close to me. I called my husband, my mother, and my supervisor where I was supposed to do the assessments for the day to tell them the big news. I immediately canceled my day and headed back to the airport. My husband went into fix-it mode, saying we'll get it out right away.

My mother took a little longer for the truth to set in. She kept saying, "No, you don't." I had to keep repeating that I do. Once reality hit her, she called everyone she knew. I really didn't want the entire planet knowing the intimate details of my life.

I headed back to the car rental place. The guy looked at me like, "Returning already?" I was tempted to say, "Yeah, breast cancer kind of cuts trips short."

But I refrained. When I was on the shuttle on the way back to the airport, my brother called. At this point, I knew that my mother had called everyone. My brother is not a man of many words—unless he has had plenty of vodka—so that was an interesting conversation. I would be having this conversation with not only those around me, but with myself, for a very long time.

I got to the airport and was able to get on a flight right away. As soon as I was seated on the plane, I ordered a glass of wine. I would have had a whole lot more than one, but I didn't want the flight attendants thinking I was an alcoholic getting plastered at 11 in the morning.

Once I landed, I went right to my primary care doctor's office. By now, the whole office must have known that "she is the girl with cancer," because the front desk guy said they had been expecting me. The medical assistant got me right back, and the doctor came in. She again mentioned that she looked up my type of cancer and couldn't find anything about it.

Seriously?

I'm going to die, and you don't even know what to blame in my obituary. Very comforting. I started to zone out, not comprehending anything that she said after that point. I was instead Charlie Brown listening to his teachers "wah wah wah wah."

She gave me the name of three breast surgeons that she

recommends to everyone, and then offered me Xanax. I guess that's the way a physician comforts. I'm not usually one for Xanax, but when it's offered in a situation like this, I figured, "What the hell?"

When I left the doctor's office, I got the "oh you poor thing, you're going to die" hug and went right to Target to get the Xanax filled. At this time, I lived in a smaller town. There is one main pharmacist that everyone knows. I hate dropping off any kind of prescriptions because I always feel like the pharmacist is judging you and thinks, "Oh, you have *that.*"

I was going to use the cancer card when filling up for these drugs that are scripted for anxiety and panic disorders, but then I didn't feel like going into a big explanation.

Once I got home, my husband, as usual, moved into crisis mode, and again assured me that we would get it "all out." My parents were far away in Illinois and were freaking out. Mom freaks out about the littlest of things, so cancer talk was putting her into overdrive. I figured it would be best to fly her to my town so at least she could be freaking out near me.

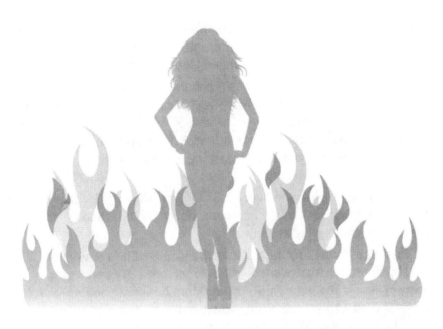

2 YOU HAVE CANCER...
NOW WHAT?

Well, if you're like me, it becomes some academic project. It was Tuesday, and I called all of the doctors on the list I was given by my PCP at Mayo Clinic. The first surgeon who is supposed to be where all of the "doctors' wives go" couldn't get me in until the following Tuesday. Okay, fine. I can wait while the cancer spreads to each area of my body.

Mayo Clinic said they could get me in on Monday, but they needed everything but my firstborn child to make it happen. That should be no problem of course. Another one of the doctors had an answering machine, and despite my message, no one called back. Finally, I called Dr. Breast Cancer Surgeon, and her assistant got me on for Thursday at 4pm. Apparently, they have a policy for those who are newly diagnosed, they take in the newly-traumatized patient and they stay overtime. She was wonderful. She spent over two hours with my husband, my mother, and me going over everything about my condition until 7pm. She even set up consults with the radiation oncologist for the next morning, an MRI for Monday, and a PET scan for Tuesday.

My schedule was full of cancer.

Her office was beautiful. Not that you should judge a physician on that, but when I used her restroom, she actually had art up that I have had up in some of my past offices. It's not very common stuff, so I knew this was a good sign. And the main walls were purple. That reminded me of one of my favorite poems, "When I'm an Old Woman, I Shall Wear Purple." And on another note, she got my jokes and sarcasm. Always a good thing.

In the meantime, I was sending out my pathology reports to the directors of the major cancer centers in California and Arizona. I was shocked because I got immediate responses. The director of the UCLA/Revlon center offered to see me as soon as she got back from vacation, which was May 24, 2010. Sorry, I was not waiting that long.

Another researcher at UC Irvine suggested that with the rarity of the cancer, she would do chemo first to see what protocol works first. Are you kidding me? With that kind of reasoning, I could just cut off my left breast altogether, using a common kitchen knife like that guy who was trapped between stones when hiking and cut off his hand. Finally, the last surgeon's assistant called and said that she could fit me in sometime in June. This was being treated like a sinus infection.

I read one article where a woman with my type of cancer had the tumor double in size in a matter of two weeks. Reading the blogs is not a good idea, by the way. The surgeon whom "all the doctors' wives" go to asked for me come to her office before my Tuesday appointment to pick up some information and a DVD to watch before the appointment. I drove over to the office. I walked into the waiting room, and it kind of creeped me out. I have been in general surgeon's offices—male general surgeons' offices—that looked better.

Seeing that surgeons are mostly in the operating room, they don't usually spend a lot on their follow-up office. But this was ridiculous. I certainly didn't think that I would be getting a spa robe or a silky poncho to wear before seeing the doctor. I took the information nonetheless, being the polite girl I am—instead of saying what I was thinking: "Really, this is a breast surgeon's office? I mistook it for a urology office." I imagined my father here. Needless to say, after meeting Dr. Fabulous Breast Surgeon with the purple walls, familiar art and spending two hours with me, I went with her.

In the meantime, what does one do while waiting for the next move? This is where the wine and cheese outings start, knowing that those times will be limited after surgery.

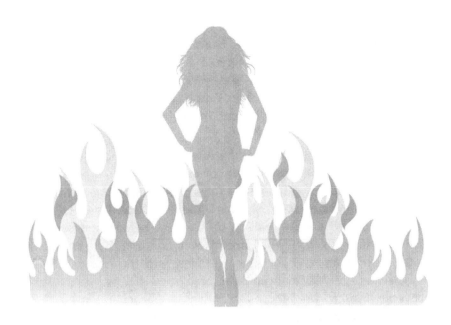

3 THE HAIRCUT
May 2010

Dr. Breast Cancer Surgeon, on the first famous night that I met her, mentioned in the moments before I walked out of the door of her office, what my new look routine should be. Since "children are involved," she suggested, I should really think about cutting my hair a little bit at a time so that they are not shocked when I have none during chemo. I can't remember the last time I cut my hair. I have been trying to grow it out since I was a teenager. As a matter of fact, a couple of weeks ago, I was ready to order a product that makes your hair "longer and stronger" from an ad I heard on the radio. Ironically, this same ad states that the product works especially well and is safe for cancer patients after chemotherapy.

So, the hair predicament.

I have several thoughts on the hair dilemma that cancer has exposed to me to. First of all, I do desperately need a haircut. My ends are bad. My split ends are splitting. I have no shape to my hair, and for most of the month prior to this, I have been sporting a ponytail—trying not to overstress it by blow drying or curling it so it will grow. My hair is not the greatest texture, but at least I still have it. However, there is part of

13

me that tells me that if I actually cut my hair, I'm submitting myself to the whims of cancer, admitting its control over my life, and that I will then have to go through chemo. I'm still enjoying my denial phase, that this is really a bad dream, or a bad *Lifetime* movie that will soon end when the news comes on at 10pm. Getting my haircut means that I'm with the program; a program I have no voice really in scheduling or producing.

At this point, I'm still hopeful that the shmuck pathologist who first diagnosed my biopsy as metaplastic carcinoma mixed up the vials. I was waiting for the apology call and the relief that would come with it. This became my ultimate fantasy. My plan is to rejoice that this was all a bad dream, a sort of wake-up call to be a better person and savor the moment before suing the hell out of everyone and their brother for missed work, pain, and suffering. Perhaps with the money, I'll earn some new leisure skills that can be accomplished NOT by sitting in a bed recovering from surgery. More like sitting on a beach in Hawaii. Then I will really go wild and buy a whole new set of white t-shirts and khaki and black pants or shorts. After all, some of mine are getting worn. This was now my dream.

I spoke to my aunt who recently went through breast cancer, surgery, and chemo about the hair issue. She stated that she, too, was trying to grow it out before it had happened to her, but rather than slowly chopping it away, she got it cut, and then my uncle shaved it for her. This saved her from letting it fall out on its own. Since her hair has grown back, she has offered to send me all of the scarves, turbans and hats that she used during chemo. One would think this is a fabulously kind gesture from one cancer patient or survivor to another (I'm not sure of the lingo that is used at this point. According to my oncologist, there is a shift when you call yourself patient versus survivor. I assume I'm still the patient status). Yet somehow, having her send me all of this stuff in a big box does not seem very appealing. I mean, don't get me wrong, I love getting packages in the mail. As a matter of fact, the UPS guy knows us personally now for all the orders my husband and I make. Between what I order and what my husband orders, we are on a first-name basis with UPS, USPS, and FedEx delivery teams. I just cannot gather up the excitement of getting a box of "cancer patient" stuff.

Did you know that this stuff has its own little industry? They have complete catalogs for this stuff. When I was at my breast surgeon's office, I was looking through her magazines as I was waiting and there was a catalog with women on the front with turbans and brightly colored hats. I picked it up and thought, "Hmm, this is an interesting cover for a magazine." Low and behold, it was a catalog from the American Cancer Society with a variety of turbans, scarves, hats and even earrings and stuff that one can adorn their bald head. I had no idea. I guess it makes sense to have them all in one place so you don't have to go looking for them. I felt the same way I did when my great aunt died, and I was at the funeral home looking around and they, too, had their own catalogs and magazines for funeral home stuff. "Best embalming fluid ever." and "You'll ride in style with our hearse accessories." Who knew?

So, instead of cutting my hair right way, I decided to color it blonder than usual. I just colored it a while ago but thought I might as well singe the hell out of it. Plus, coloring it and not cutting is a way of dodging that I'm with the program. I also figure that if I do get the apology call, I can add the price of the box of color to the settlement, along with labor, of course. With my new plan of resistance, my mom got me a box of ultra-light blonde. I put it all over my head, like I usually do, because heaven forbid that I actually take the time or the money to have someone else color it. Well, once again, coloring it myself turns most of it orange or as my mother would say, "chicken shit yellow." I'm not deterred. The ponytail is still an option.

Since the surgery was postponed and I had some extra time, I decided I could at least get a trim. I needed it anyway and I don't have to cut it all off. Dr. Breast Cancer Surgeon said only a couple of inches to start. I've gotten a couple of inches off lots of times so obviously this does not mean I'm admitting I have cancer. My hair is about to my bra line at this point, which interestingly I won't need either soon. Besides, I'm in limbo, and I'm having no luck with the leisure skill goals on my treatment plan.

I decided to go to Cost Cutters down the road from my house on my way to Target. That way it really feels more like just a regular errand, not some major life decision related to my real-life nightmare. Not only that, but I'm not going to pay a lot of money on a haircut if it's all going to fall out soon. Let's be practical.

I parked the car and walked into the shop. Of course, on a Friday afternoon with no cars in the parking lot, there is only one stylist in the whole place who is working on a tween in a Hannah Montana shirt. And of course, the hairstylist has that one streak in her hair that looks like she and the other girls were experimenting on each other in their downtime. I sign my name on the log and the hairdresser tells me it will just be about 10 minutes because the other girl went to the bank.

Ten minutes. Okay, I can wait 10 minutes. After all, I need to pick out a style, a "medium length" style from one of the many hairstyling books in the waiting room that look like they are from 1970. Then panicked, I remember that the last time I went to a discount haircutting place and asked for something other than a trim, I got a perplexed look from the 12-year-old behind the counter. She told me that a new style was extra.

Whatever, it all *might* fall out soon anyway. After all, even if I do give into the fact I have cancer, maybe I will be the one person whose hair doesn't fall out. I'm sitting there and the stylist gets done with the tween, and then her brother jumps in the chair. At this point, I'm thinking, "Doesn't she know I have cancer? Maybe I should tell her. Should I play the 'cancer card' to get ahead in line?" I decide against it and walk out, saying that I'm going to do some shopping and then come back—*maybe*.

I get back into the car to drive the fifty yards to Target. There's just something about Target. My mom says that I'm there so much that I should have the bull's eye tattooed on my butt. When you have two little kids and you can get shredded cheese, the latest movies, and a bra in the same place, why would you go anywhere else? We needed the usual at the house: pull-ups, juice, Diet Coke, and bottled water. My mother suggested that with the surgery and chemo coming up, we should all start using Purell on a regular basis.

The kids need to also learn the fine art of washing hands the waterless way. I load up the cart with the super-giant Target brand bottle of antibacterial instant hand sanitizer, along with various other sizes, including the handy travel bottle. I get up to the counter with all of these sanitizers, and the woman at the register gives me a strange look. I say with a smile, "I'm going to try to get obsessive-compulsive disorder."

Once again, I get the blank deer-in-the-headlight look. Good humor wasted on humorless people.

I get back into the car and think of whatever errands I can think of. The bank? The grocery store? Maybe I can sneak in a twist ice cream cone from McDonald's. No one will ever know about it, because I'm actually driving around town with no kids in the car. After exhausting my mind with potential errands to run, there was still that dreaded haircut. I figured I might as well drive by. Cancer diagnosis or not, chicken shit yellow hair is a not a look to walk around with. Sure enough, this time when I pull in to the shop, four stylists are standing outside smoking. I guess the tweens went home, and the skunk-streaked hairdresser is still there along with someone else, who seemed to be the hair dummy for a training session on Color 101 gone totally wrong. Do I dare walk in and declare my cancer through a new hairstyle? I began to distract myself with the salon pecking order and whose dummy I will be. Will I get skunk head, blue hair, old lady who is working one day a week to get out of the house, or, wait, there is one girl with her hair a normal color and not in some crazy style.

The stars aligned, and I get Normal Girl.

"Just a trim?" There it is, the question to which my answer will declare my submission to the illness.

"No, I've just been diagnosed with breast cancer, and my doctor suggested I start getting it cut slowly so I don't shock my kids as clumps fall." Okay, I didn't say that out loud.

Instead I say, "Maybe a couple of inches off."

Normal Girl sits me in her chair and starts to comb out my hair. She hesitates for a moment, like all hair stylists do when they notice that someone bought a five-dollar box of hair dye and did their own color.

"How long ago did you color your hair?"

"Not too long ago," I replied, embarrassed.

Again, a freakishly nice person, she tells me that she can get the "brassiness" out by applying a toner. I believe that is the polite way of saying, "Dang, you really screwed up your hair."

She was so excited about it because she had just done the same thing to her friend's hair and it looked "awesome." I didn't want to dampen her mood, so I said yes. Besides, I wasn't sure if I was going to announce I had cancer, it will soon be irrelevant, since this haircut after all was my announcement to myself.

Next comes the small talk. This is usually a dreaded time anyway because inevitably, I'm asked what I do for a living. I usually get two different types of reactions when I say I'm psychologist. The first reaction I get is that which a person shares more details than I ever wanted to know about the person's life and their sister's son who has some type of disorder with a bunch of letters like ESP or something. Or, I get a look like, "You, yeah right," and then silence.

Normal Girl didn't launch into this usual line of questioning right away because she was obviously excited to be doing something other than the usual men's haircut with clippers. Even Skunk Head Girl walked by and exclaimed, "Oooh, you're doing color?!"

I would like to add that this trip to the salon counts toward my leisure skill objectives on my treatment plan. Normally, I would never had taken the time to sit there to do a cut and color had it not been planned out and time carved out accordingly. This was a rare spontaneity on my part, and I wasn't even watching the clock. I simply did my own cognitive exercises, telling myself that it was okay to take the time. Yes, even psychologists have issues.

For example, I began to think why is it that in order to get beautified you have to suffer through some ugliness. Normal Girl put goop on my hair so that my hair and the goop were pasted to my head. It looked like I had no hair. I tried not to think about it and started the small talk on my own. Apparently Normal Girl is not the sharpest knife in the drawer. She proceeded to tell me how she now has a stalker. She was dating a guy for three months before she realized he had paranoid schizophrenia and that the FBI guys he was talking about weren't real.

And since I was a psychologist, I should understand, she told me. I laughed and said, "Molly, looks like he had some red flags. Might want to avoid schizophrenics as part of your dating pool." At this point, she looked up and said, "How did you know my name?"

I just knew at this point my hair was going to come out green. "Molly, it's on your license and all over your mirror." She even had a sticky note on her mirror that said *Remember to go to the bank on Monday.* She commented that it works great because all of her customers then remind her to go to the bank on Mondays.

Okay. Normal Girl is now Not-So-Normal Girl. Yeah, I don't think Not-So-Normal Girl could handle me telling her that I have cancer, and the whole point of the haircut is to start the slow, painful process of going from long stringy hair, to medium style, to pixie cut to no hair. She has enough problems of her own. Getting to work might be one of them. I just couldn't push her over the edge like that.

Once again, I had to use my psychological powers for good and not evil. Instead of making comments that I knew she would not understand for my own enjoyment, I actually talked to her about dating strategies—like being pickier or maybe using the internet. I went into therapist-patient mode. Surprisingly, or really shockingly, this attractive 36-year-old woman (yes, at some point she told me her age and more details than I needed) has never sent an email out in her life and has no idea how to use the computer, and yes, she said that out loud. As a matter of fact, her mother told her that if she would take a computer course, she would buy her a laptop. I guess her family recognizes she is on the left side of the bell curve.

Not-So-Normal Girl started to trim my hair. She actually did a great job. I got about four inches cut off—still enough hair to have a nice ponytail. And believe it or not, the color was no longer orange, but a really great shade of blonde with nice highlights. Molly might not know what Google is, but she can do hair. We all have our gifts. I started to look in the mirror, actually admiring the final presentation—I paid extra for her to "blow it out." Then it hit me as I was admiring my hair, I finally take the time to get my haircut from a discount haircutting place no less, only to know that I might not have it in a couple of months. There is always the possibility that I will get that apology call, and I can add this to the settlement. Shit. I finally had a decent color and cut.

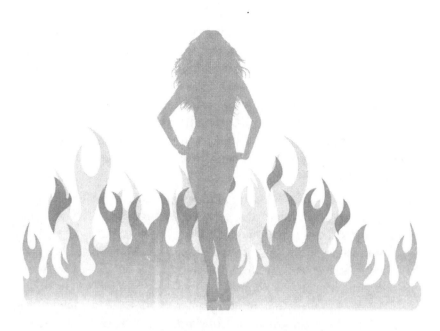

4 IT'S VERY REAL

May 14-17, 2010

Unfortunately, I didn't get a call from the path lab stating that they switched the slides. If they can switch babies in the hospital, why couldn't my destiny be switched? I've been buying lottery tickets, I mean, there has to be a balance somewhere. The reality of CANCER is getting real.

The surgeon I picked has so far been wonderful. She has set everything up, and her office gets everything authorized. Apparently if I stay in-network, after my deductible almost everything should be paid for. I won't have to strip for dollars afterward to pay for all of this—a breast-less stripper probably only gets spare change—not the full dollar. Or customers with odd fetishes.

On Friday, I met with Dr. Radiation Oncologist. He met with me for over two hours—dang—again. What's with the freakishly nice people I'm dealing with, and why did they come at a time like this and not the normal days? By the end, he gave me his cell phone number in case I needed it. He is originally from Wisconsin so he has that going for him— I'm from Illinois and went to college in Kenosha, Wisconsin. He's even been to the bar where I used to hang out in college. We shared cheese curd stories. The digression is obvious, but the comfort in being in a relevant environment as I battled this out brought enough meaning to me to push forward.

His practice is literally pioneering new radiation techniques. One of the partners invented a modified radiation technique that decreases the amount of time that radiation treatments are needed. It's now a standard of care across the country. Dr. Radiation Oncologist also studied at the University of Arizona Tucson, which apparently is one of the leading cancer centers in the nation.

Things were becoming more relative.

Dr. Radiation Oncologist said that he really cannot say whether or not I will need radiation until he sees the pathology reports after the surgery. Studies are inconclusive about the need for radiation with this type of cancer. It depends on how big the tumor is, if it's in the lymph nodes, and how close it's to the chest wall. So far, what I've read from blogs states that this type of cancer responds well to radiation. The big outcome of this meeting was that I will have to wait to have reconstructive surgery. It makes sense that reconstruction can only occur after a full on demolition.

Having breast reconstruction at the time of the mastectomy could complicate the radiation treatment later, this is fine with me and the surgeon. This means that the first surgery will have slightly less recovery time than a mastectomy with reconstruction. I might be able to wear a prosthetic after surgery. Do you know they sell those at Nordstrom? The industry was actually doing that well. The good news is that if you ask to see my new breasts after the surgery, I can take one out and hand it to you.

So, after this appointment, I headed over to have an MRI. The freakishly nice people were swarming about. I mean, I'm adorable, but no one knows me here! Even the MRI tech spent time with me. I had the MRI after they gave me a spa robe to change into, books and a glitter pink breast cancer pin. I hate to say it, but the pink was getting sickening.

I went to have a PET scan of my whole body to see if the cancer has spread anywhere. The PET scan was at 11:30am. No sugar and no "white foods" 24 hours before the test, and then no food—only water—6 hours before the test. What seemingly starts off as a good diet, becomes a hunger strike. You can just imagine how crabby I was not eating for that long. Apparently, the radioactive isotope they send through your veins is to see if there is cancer. Cancer absorbs sugars differently—so you have to avoid all sugar for 24 hours. I did cheat and have a glass of wine on Sunday night—but then drank about a gallon of water to make sure it was out of my system. It paid off. The MRI tech took my blood sugar and said it was the lowest that he had ever seen and that I MUST have really followed the diet. If only I could cheat the cancer that easily.

I had to "rest" my muscles for 24 hours before the test as well. My husband joked, "Looks like we'll have to forgo that five-mile hike we usually take on Sundays." This new chapter in my life was the hike of a lifetime.

The whole test took about two hours. Of course, I had to ask how really overweight people get through the big tube. I was that kind of person and I do weight loss surgery evaluations for a living. The tech told me that it's very uncomfortable for them—with that freakishly friendly smile, of course. At the end of the PET scan, there were cookies. Praise the Lord, the hunger strike was over! Again, the tech was super nice and put together a stack of four cookies for me in a bag—just for me. Ahhhh! The little things.

Since I'm not having reconstruction during the surgery, I don't need to meet with the plastic surgery guy yet. My surgeon also said that I can wait to meet with the oncologist until after surgery so I don't get overloaded with information. However, she did call the oncologist when I was in her office to check about hair loss with the kind of chemo I will need after surgery. I started admitting to myself the reality of cancer, and, as extreme as this all was becoming to me and what was once a normal life, I was thinking about dying my hair purple. Seeing that I only wear white, black, and beige—that might be a little wild for me.

I called Dr. Breast Cancer Surgeon's office after the PET scan to see if there was anything else I needed to do or anyone else I needed to see. I spoke to the office receptionist, and she said she would get back to me by the end of the day. Now get this—the doctor—Dr. Breast Cancer Surgeon—actually called me back herself. I feel like I'm in the twilight zone, what with doctors calling me back themselves.

She said that the PET scan came back clear except for something strange on my breast plate. She thinks it's probably nothing. However, the radiologist who read the MRI was concerned about something she saw that may indicate lymph node activity, which, apparently was not seen on the PET scan. As the doctors shot ideas back and forth, I had another appointment with the MRI radiologist to have a special ultrasound at the kind time of 7:30am. If anything weird is found, then I will have a biopsy of the lymph node immediately following. To be frank, all the cancer blogs I've read basically noted that this would suck. This kind of cancer goes into the chest wall and into the lungs more often than the lymph system. If it's in the lymph nodes, then Dr. Breast Cancer Surgeon says that her surgical strategy will be slightly different.

With all these different tests, I was back to being a student. I was online researching everything I could.

Finally, I meet with Dr. Breast Cancer Surgeon for a pre-surgical visit on Thursday morning at 7:45 am to go over any questions or other information. She reflected her positive outlook despite all this, and announced that the surgery is tentatively scheduled for 12pm on Friday with a check-in of 10am. Despite the severity of the tests, the stress and concern, and the new hairstyle I had done, it was all for an outpatient surgery. Yes, that's right. Because there was no reconstruction, there would be no need to stay overnight unless some complications or pain confined me to the hospital bed. I thought about milking it.

However, the goal is to get you out of the hospital as soon as possible so you're not exposed to anything like MRSA. Dr. Breast Cancer Surgeon said that they would not be doing much at the hospital other than what I would be doing at home. Of course, I mentioned that at the hospital, they would be cooking for me, bringing me my meals, and I would have a buzzer to summon "staff" at a moment's notice. She was not impressed.

I'm trying to stay positive. I honestly anticipate faltering a bit after surgery, and I assume that is when this will all hit me. The books I'm reading say that surgery is the easy part. In the meantime, I have a new three-ring binder with dividers and a place for results, records, and business card holders, any excuse to buy paper products to keep me from thinking about post-op.

I plan on working as much as I can from home to keep my sanity. I have not yet mastered the art of leisure skills, although I'm sure I have it on a treatment plan somewhere. Downtime will be difficult for me. It's already obvious I'm thinking too much.

And the thoughts only surge as I find out that surgery has been postponed until next Wednesday, May 19. The good news is that apparently I've been the talk of the town with the surgeons and oncologists. The guy who wrote the textbook on radiation said there is probably a less than one percent chance I will need radiation. Also, the results of the lymph node biopsy were negative, thus making it even less likely that I will need radiation. As a result, we can actually go ahead with the reconstruction at the same time as the surgery. This will eliminate another surgery down the line. However, recovery will obviously be a little rougher.

This was all good news; relatively speaking, of course. I'm off to the plastic surgeon and the oncologist. This delay gives me another weekend to hit the vino before surgery and that can't be a bad thing, right?

■

My adventures in Doctor Appointment Land started at 7:30am and ended somewhere after 5pm. My first appointment was with the breast surgeon, this was supposed to be the "pre-op" appointment before surgery today. However, since there is such a tiny chance that I'll need radiation, Dr. Breast Cancer Surgeon really encouraged me to go for the reconstruction at the same time as the surgery. As I mentioned yesterday, this means postponing the surgery so I could meet with the plastic surgeon.

Obviously, this was good news, but after having myself psyched to have major surgery today, it was a bit of an emotional rollercoaster. My life was at a stop-go pattern, and being at the whims of the doctors, who obviously knew best, was not easy for my mind to grasp. Not to mention that the recovery time and the hospital stay for this two-for-one surgery will be longer. Doctor Appointment Land had taken its toll.

I was hopping from one place to the next, awaiting news and decisions from those who would seemingly rescue me. Dr. Breast Cancer Surgeon was amazing and made appointments for me to see both the plastic surgeon and the oncologist. Who has that kind of skill to get appointments with specialists on the same day? Either this surgeon is that good, or my adorableness really shines even more than I thought! Maybe it was the new haircut. Given the situation, I will go with the latter since the former might mean urgency.

The next stop of the day was the plastic surgeon's office. My father flew into town Wednesday night and decided that he wanted to tag along to the appointments. Of course, he waited in the waiting room when I went in. Although I'm completely grateful that my parents are here for support, I have to tell you that sitting next to your parents at almost 40 years old in an office with glass sculptures of breasts everywhere is a little awkward. Of course, on the way over to the appointment, I mentioned to my dad that I didn't remember him EVER coming to a doctor's appointment with us when I was younger!

For those of you wondering if my plastic surgeon was going to look something like Drs. McDreamy or McSteamy from *Grey's Anatomy*, you're sadly mistaken. Although my surgeon is not like Derek Sheppard, he was completely wonderful and empathetic. Again, he spent a huge amount of time with me and my mom. I saw pictures of his work, and I have to say all of the women looked better and "rejuvenated", which was his word. My word would be they looked "perkier" after surgery. As I've seen lots of plastic surgery work with the weight loss surgery people from work, I have to say he's pretty good.

He started to explain the surgery and how the expanders will work. He then said that he fashions the nipple and tattoos it himself. I asked him if he also did tattoo parties on the side. I actually said that out loud. He didn't quite get my humor. I don't think he has seen a patient like me for a while. Apparently, he and I will be big buddies after the surgery because he has to fill up the expanders several times, and then I need another surgery after that.

Before leaving his office, I gave him a list of things I needed him to do before the surgery—not attend any drug rep parties the night before, I want to be first on the schedule so he won't be tired after working on someone else, no staying up late the night before my surgery, to eat a good breakfast, no fights with his wife the day before or the day of, and my list of conditions continued. Again, he looked at me somewhat puzzled and said, "I guess you know a little bit about surgery."

The final stop of the day was the oncologist's office. I have heard a lot of good things about this particular doctor from my research and the other physicians I have spoken with. The radiation guy said she was very upbeat, funny, and "touchy-feely." Dr. Breast Cancer Surgeon said that if she had to have chemo herself, she would only go to her. I walked into her office and thought I was walking into a spa. There is a waterfall, gorgeous decorative use of the room, and the serenity I was supposed to be looking for during my leisure time. The guy at the reception desk was of the freakishly friendly. He immediately lets me and my parents know that there is a "snack" area with water, tea, lattes, and healthy munchies if we want any. He also wanted to let me know that they are expanding their services to include massages, yoga, and organic manicures and pedicures. What was this place? At this point all I needed was Brad Pitt to come out and offer me some chocolate. This place was that nice. Of course, as he is saying this, one woman walks past me in the waiting room all dressed up with high heel sandals, a dress, full makeup, and jewelry. I turned to my mom and said, "Damn, am I going to have to dress up for chemo?" It seemed like chemotherapy was going to be a special affair.

Finally, I, along with my parents, am whisked back to a private room. As we walk to the room, we pass several large La-Z-Boy chairs that overlook a peaceful scene over the desert. One lady was surrounded by her girlfriends as she is hooked up to an IV. We pass a little area with wigs, scarves, jewelry, flip-flops, and other ornaments. The medical assistant invites us to "look around while we wait" if we want. Once in the room, there is another La-Z-Boy and a television to watch while we wait for the doctor. I'm telling you, this makes my office look like a dump.

Dr. Oncologist, a petite woman, floats into the room calmly and with purpose, like a Greek goddess on a cloud. She is extremely cheerful, warm and also shares that element of being freakishly nice. Her vocabulary set is one that consists of "honey", "sweetie", and "love". Dr. Oncologist asks me what I know about my cancer and the possible treatment. Of course, I take out my pink three-ring notebook and start pulling out research I have outlined and email responses I have received from the directors of the University of Arizona Cancer Care Center, a major breast cancer researcher at UCI, and the director of UCLA's Revlon/Breast Clinic.

She proceeds to tell me that it looks like my cancer is not entirely "Triple Negative" because my progesterone receptor came back positive and the HER-2 (I think that's what she said—and I thought psychologists had a lot of abbreviations) is still pending. Apparently, this is good news because then several medications can be used that have been proven to be effective. However, this will again be pending the final pathology report. She also states that she has worked with metaplastic cancer in the past, which is good.

She was very hopeful, but again gave me a lot of information that I could in no way repeat. I have no idea what she said, but my mother, being an actual nurse, wrote it all down. The doctor was so positive about the whole process of chemotherapy and the drugs that are given to get rid of side effects. However, my hairstyle was doomed—that is one side effect that won't go away with a pill. I kind of felt like I was back in the twilight zone. Have you ever had anybody tell you how great something is going to be when it really involves jumping off a cliff? That's what the twilight zone feels like. Of course, the psychologist in me knew that she was "working on my mind psychologically", since studies indicate that patients who have a positive attitude and are hopeful have better outcomes. So, I just went with it. Better than having some old guy tell me, "Well, not sure if this is going to work, but we'll try."

I asked her, "How do they tell if the chemo is working or what objective markers they go by?"

What she said merely revealed that the twilight zone had no form of gravity or laws for that matter.

"There is no way to tell."

They take certain markers in the blood but nothing that says, *Hey we got all the cancer! Hey, chemo is working!* Now I know how patients must feel when they read my consent that says, "There is no guarantee that therapy will help."

The twilight zone was winning and I was floating around in the mess of it.

At the end, she gave me a big hug and then sent me off to have my blood level checked. Did I mention the hugging? All of the doctors I have met give hugs—with the exception of the plastic surgeon guy—which I'm totally fine with a no-hugging policy in that situation. I'm not the hugging type. I can count the number of patients I have hugged after a session on one hand. I'm really more of the *boundaries-in-place, pat on the back* kind of girl. In the twilight zone, there were no boundaries, and this is an adjustment for me. I guess since I just walked around their offices topless for a better part of the appointments, they may feel some sort of closeness that comes with nakedness.

After my adventures in Doctor Appointment Land, I got home and crashed. Then Dr. Breast Cancer Surgeon called me at about 7pm, with the promptness no one would expect of a doctor outside of the twilight zone, to let me know that the surgery date might not be Wednesday but

Friday, but she is not sure. They're trying to coordinate her schedule, the plastic surgeon's time and the OR time. It might not even be at the original hospital we talked about. I'm in limbo now as the twilight zone flips on its head. The surgery could be anytime next week.

Apparently this is all good, again, relatively speaking. I mean, before May 4th, my big disappointment was not getting the parking spot closest the store.

■

When I thought that my surgery was scheduled for Friday, I went out and bought a bunch of See's Candy. I mean, who wouldn't? I bought two boxes of wonderful chocolate creams. The idea was that I would have some now, before the surgery, because I anticipate that after the surgery I'm only going to crave high protein, low-carb shakes that the weight loss surgery patients are supposed to drink.

Now that the surgery has been postponed until next week—what day, I don't know—there are two boxes of chocolates sitting on the countertop. I think I'm almost through one. That was not the plan. So now I'm going to see how long I can exist on just wine and chocolate and the occasionally carbohydrate just so I don't get sick from eating too much chocolate. Not much of a healthy eating strategy to be as "healthy as I can before surgery." I know. But damn, it tastes so good to be reckless.

■

The surgery date has been tentatively set for Friday, May 21, 2010 at 10:30am. I say "tentatively" because I feel a bit out of the loop since I haven't seen a doctor now for about four days. Once upon a time, I had not been to the doctor's in four years. The silence was troubling, and I had to call the doctor's office to make sure that they didn't forget about me. They didn't. It's on the schedule.

I'm attempting to get as many work-related items as I can done before I'm immobile for a while. I also thought about starting a rigorous exercise program this morning but, after I called the doctor's office, I figured, why start? I've been working on my arms, hoping that I can have Arnold Schwarzenegger arms by Friday. That might be kind of tough since I'm doing it without any weights.

I did get the case of protein shakes today in anticipation for the cravings I'm hoping to have after surgery. I figured if I have protein shakes, I'm bound to improve my healing process and have the added benefit of losing a couple of pounds.

But who was I kidding? From the chocolate to whatever my diet would be after the surgery, the stress from such situations was sending my brain back on that rollercoaster. While I'm usually a fabulous multi-tasker, this last week has got me realizing what dementia might feel like. I left the house without my phone yesterday. I never do that. I actually drove around town for a while without it and even when I finally got home to get it, I still couldn't find it. I literally had no recollection of where I had put it. It turns out it was in my son's room on his dresser. I must have left it there while I was trying to get him ready, and no, I had not been drinking. When there is a mass in your breast, weighing on your heart, and burdening your brain, the tendencies, routines, memory, and strength all become imbalanced.

As I'm getting ready for nursing home status, I've been going through a list of things to remember with my parents and husband. Things like the last week of school for the kids is next week and they have parties, so I've been assigned things to bring. My daughter has playgroup. This stress-related dementia is not only affecting me, but those around me. My mom says to me, "You'll need to write down for me all of the doctors' offices so we know where we are going when we take you to the aftercare appointments." I turn to her and said, "You know, I'll still be able to speak after surgery." My dad, who usually doesn't say much, says, "Yeah, I don't think they're sewing her mouth shut." The brain is just not firing all at once.

When I was out getting my protein shakes at Costco today, who else is out shopping but the radiologist who did my original ultrasound and biopsy. Now remember, this is a woman who should be on the World Poker Tour because she had the best poker face of anyone I know. Talk about an awkward situation. Of course, I couldn't tell if she recognized me or not. I thought about taking off my shirt and introducing myself that way, since that's how she last saw me. How does one even start that conversation? "Hi, Dr. Radiologist, so good to see you. I don't know if you remember me, but you were sticking a huge needle in my breast just last week. Shop at Costco often?"

I mean, as a breast radiologist, she must get that a lot, right? I decided against it. My parents were with me and talking about breasts in front of my dad, which was still uncomfortable. Introducing Dr. Radiologist to my dad might have been indeed uncomfortable. *Hey Dad, this is Dr. Radiologist. She diagnosed me with cancer.* Yeah. That wasn't going to work.

As we walked around Costco, the variety of products and the sight of my doctor made me realize all the different types of breasts. Now that I will get new ones, I find myself looking around like I'm shopping for a new outfit. "Wow that girl has a nice rack. A little big in case I want to do that triathlon in the future."

Then there are the rag magazines highlighting Heidi Montag's FFF chest. And it looks like Kate Hudson also expanded her dimensions. Of course, I think my husband is voting for Heidi Montag replicas. When my aunt had her reconstruction, she asked for exactly the same size. I'm tending toward her decision, but then I have to decide the size before kids or after kids. Breasts were always changing, and that was life. I went up about a cup size after the darlings were born. I read an article where Pamela Anderson switches out sizes like she changes underwear.

It makes you think that maybe you should be able to rotate them like people who have no legs, or like tires on a car. They have their running legs and then their "everyday legs." I'll have to ask my short, balding Asian plastic surgeon the choices the industry has made available.

5 THE NIGHT BEFORE

May 20, 2010

The night before the rest of your life, what exactly do you do? The countdown has begun. I got the final call from the surgeon's office and the hospital that the surgery is indeed scheduled for Friday, May 21, 2010 at 10:30am with a check-in time of 8:30am. Did you get that? A "check-in" time of 8:30am. Did I mention that most of these places where I've been for tests have "check-in" times? It's like I'm checking into a great hotel or a five-star luxury resort. I love these little mind tricks. It's as if the whole situation is made more pleasant with a "check-in" time, the spa robe, and the snack area.

They're not fooling me. I'm on to them. I'm a psychologist after all.

When the nurse from the hospital called, she went over my medical history and what I should and shouldn't bring the day of the surgery. She mentioned that I will have to have someone drive me home. That one was obvious. The list went on. I can't wear my contacts or makeup. Okay, contacts I get, but I have not left the house without at least mascara on since 1984. This situation is getting rougher by the minute and the list got longer. She told me I had to wash my hair and use no hair products. Again, I can't remember the last time I washed my hair without putting some kind of mousse or gel in it. Frankly, without makeup and hair products, I'm worried that the surgeons I met last week won't recognize me. At least the short, balding Asian guy took pictures of my breasts. Hopefully, he will have those as a reference. However, I think that walking into the hospital topless is frowned upon.

Speaking of Dr. Plastic Surgeon (you'll have to excuse my random thoughts—I've been a little disjointed lately), I was wondering what pair of breasts does he visualize when he is operating? Think about it. When you work on something three-dimensional, generally the way the mind works is that you create a picture in your mind as a blueprint. Even when you rearrange a room, you have a vision in your head first. So whose breasts is this guy working from—a girl he got a peek of in college? Or, knowing my luck, he has an old lady fetish. Let's keep our fingers crossed and hope for the former.

Speaking of breasts, my breasts in particular, I have been reading in some of my "How to Survive Breast Cancer" books that some women have a goodbye party for their breasts or something like that the night before the surgery. They take pictures, talk to their breasts, and make a scrapbook project called "My Breasts, My Friends"—stuff like that. I won't be doing that. In general, I'm not a sentimental person. I don't save napkins from "special dinners." I don't have a special drawer of keepsakes. At Christmas time, I don't spend time reminiscing about where I got an ornament or about Christmases in the past. If it was up to me, I would have one of those trees that folds up with all the fixings on it like an umbrella and store it. Instead, I was thinking about how much wine I could drink before midnight—this, of course, being the cut-off before I'm "NPO" before surgery—nothing taken by mouth—no water, no gum, no candy, no pills—nothing. I figure that if I have too much wine, I will be unconscious for a good part of the hangover and I will be getting good drugs and a saline drip—the perfect solution to a hangover.

Again, not being as sentimental as I once was, I really hope that all of the cards I have been getting offering encouragement and support are not a sign that I'm at death's door. I really do not plan on knocking on that door for quite a while. I mean, who would remember what day to put out the garbage? I guess being a "caretaker" for a living makes it a little hard for me to be cared for myself. But I will admit that as a working mother (as I'm sure many of you can appreciate) I'm fantasizing about being waited on and not cleaning or cooking for a while. I have to laugh. When I have psychiatrically hospitalized women in the past, that is the one thing they say that was great about it (if there is something great about being locked up in a psych ward). They all said it was wonderful that someone else took care of them. They got three square meals a day that they didn't have to cook or clean up after. No laundry. No kids yelling "Mom! Mom! Mom! Mom!"

See, now if all of the books on "How to survive breast cancer" would mention that being a bonus part of the recovery—now that makes the situation more tolerable—more so than a spa robe or a snack area!

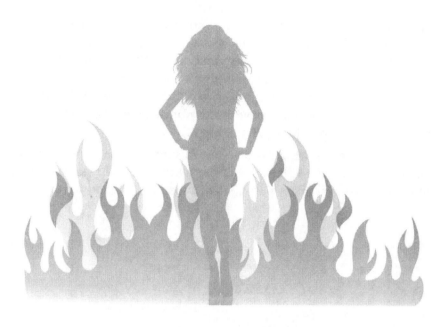

6 THE SURGERY

May 21-June 1, 2010

I've been a little busy doing nothing but taking pain medications and going to doctor's appointments. And for some reason, that makes it really hard to concentrate. Even reading a *People* magazine article is difficult. I received the final pathology report from my surgery today, but it's completely Greek. I have an appointment with the oncologist on Friday. Hopefully, she can translate it for me. I hate not understanding what I'm reading. Psychology is just a bit different than molecular biology.

The night before surgery, my mom fell down on our stairs by our pool. She *just* had knee surgery a couple of months ago. Since my surgery was the next day, she shrugged it off as a sprained ankle that was thankfully *not* on the side of her knee surgery. Since then, she has been hobbling around like a little old lady. But alas, I cannot complain since she continues to rise to the task of Mother of the Year through all of this. Once I was in the hospital, she mentioned that it was still hurting and attempted to go to the emergency room—again, since the only excitement of the days in the hospital was my countdown to the next morphine shot. Being that my surgery was in a large trauma center, every time she went down to the ER, she was going to be like the 100th person in line. Thus, she continued to wobble around.

Finally, last night she says to me that she should probably go to the ER or urgent care just in case it's broken, because, although she can walk on it, she still having some pain. So, my husband drove her to the urgent care, which was already closed. They end up at the emergency room of a less busy hospital. The ankle is actually broken, they find. The doctor looked at her like she was nuts for walking around on a broken ankle for 11 days, but that is the strength, I suppose, of being a mother. The good news is that if she would have gone into the ER the night it happened, she would have been casted and would not be able to take a shower. Since it has been 11 days since the break, they put a moon boot on it to stabilize it. And bonus, she has her own prescription of Vicodin now! I wasn't sure if I should cry or laugh.

You see, that's the thing with any ailment. Do you celebrate overcoming it, or do you lament about its impact? Being the practical person I am, I talk with my husband about when the trash is supposed to go out, what happens if I'm in the hospital longer than a night, etc. This all seemed a little tense. So, instead, we turned on the DVD player in his car and watch videos of Beyoncé singing "Single Ladies". This video really is catchy, plus, dang, how much practice went into getting all three of those girls in sync—and in high heels no less—by their male choreographer, who is also dancing in heels off to the left. Ah, the distractions.

Distractions help when the questions and conversations on the way to a mastectomy or cancer surgery seem burdensome. No one wants to bring them up. Once at the hospital, it was impossible to find a parking space. I'm glad I was mobile, because it felt like we parked a mile away. We had to check in at day surgery—even though the plan was that I was going to stay the night. The fact that I had a "check-in" time led me to believe it would be like checking into a hotel where I was greeted by name, offered bottled water, and given warm cookies. This was not the case. I had to sign my name on the HIPAA-appropriate sign-in sheets— the one with the stickers—and wait my turn.

Sitting in the waiting room was a distraction in itself. The patients were clearly identified because they all had wristbands. One woman in particular had a band on and, I swear, about three-inch nails. Now who goes into surgery with their nails three inches long? First of all, the anesthesiologist needs to see your nail beds and usually a heart rate/oxygen monitor is placed on your finger. I'm all for looking as cute as I can be, but within reason, of course. Across the way was an older couple and then a woman and her "friend". They struck up a conversation. The older man asked what the woman was having done. She hesitated for a moment, but then, like myself, I'm sure that she thought that this old coot has no manners, so what the heck. It turns out that they both had the same surgeon for their procedures, which were scheduled about an hour apart. Suddenly, they were old friends.

I kept waiting for someone to ask why I was there. I was going to tell them that I was going to have my prostate removed. Fortunately, no one asked, because by this time, my parents arrived and they would have been mortified.

Finally some woman called out my name. I jumped up like the seat was on fire. I actually registered online, so I wasn't sure what else they needed. As expected, she asked for all of the same information that I already gave online, with the exception of my magic insurance card. I got my own special bracelet with my name on it only to sit and wait some more. Once my husband and I got up, someone took our seats. We ended up sitting across from what I'm sure was seven sisters all conceived in a petri dish. They were of various ages and looked freakishly alike and not in a good way. Their noses were definitely the "before" picture in a plastic surgeon's portfolio for rhinoplasty. Of course, I can't say too much. I showed up without makeup as I was instructed. Since I look like I'm about 12 without my makeup, the nurses kept checking my wristband and yes, indeed, it said 39-year-old female every time.

Guess what? This was quite a painful surgery. I ended up in the hospital for two extra days just to manage the pain.

Interestingly, before the surgery, I asked the plastic surgeon if the surgery was going to hurt. He looked at me and said, "Some people do find it uncomfortable." For future reference, when a doctor tells you that something is going to be "uncomfortable" this actually translates into "excruciating pain like you've never known before." Whenever the nurse would come into my room to administer IV pain meds, I offered to rename my children after her.

7 POST-SURGERY

June 3, 2010

I'm trying to stay positive. However, when you go from working 24/7 to lying in bed contemplating the universe, things get a little strange to say the least.

Today, I went and visited Dr. Plastic Surgeon. I'm going to have to come up with another name for him because he is really turning out to be a good doctor and is finally getting some of my jokes. One of the reasons that I've been in so much pain is that he overfilled my expanders so my chest muscles are spastic and painful. I asked him today if everyone has this much pain because I really have a pretty high pain tolerance. I mean, when I broke my elbow, I was back to work in a couple of days. Again, he reminded me that I had a pretty major surgery and that, "It's probably my fault. I might have overfilled you, but the good news is that you will only needs about two fills." Oh joy, something to look forward to. He also took out the drains, which is nice. I was wearing them in a fanny pack that was oh-so-attractive. And yes, they did sting a little bit when he yanked them out. At least he didn't put his foot on my side for leverage to get it out.

I mentioned to my husband that when all of this is over that I want to go on a real vacation—not camping. Some place with fruity drinks with umbrellas. He jokingly said (at least I think he was joking) that the bigger the breasts, the better the vacation. Of course, he also asked if we could get a home breast pump in case we want them bigger in the future. I ignored that comment, obviously.

I'm back to my regular doctor visits now that I'm healing. I have an appointment with the oncologist tomorrow—remember the perky one (perkier than me even)—to start to look at chemo options. Then on Tuesday, I'm going down to get a second opinion about treatment for this type of tumor since it's so rare. They have also been freakishly nice getting all of my paperwork together. I really am planning on going with Dr. Perky, but I think I would be doing myself a disservice if I didn't get a second opinion given that one of the best cancer centers in the United States is only a couple of hours away.

The surgical pathology report came back for my viewing. I have no idea what it means, but my breast cancer surgeon seems to think it's all good news. Anyone out there who has a friend, enemy, or colleague who knows anything about this stuff, I will be happy to forward the report. It looks like my estrogen and HER2 receptors are negative and my progesterone receptors are 25%. Yeah, I have no idea what that means either. Hopefully, in the next couple of days the doctors that I met with can translate it for me.

Again, if you're going through something like cancer or any other exciting health issue—do NOT read the blogs (mine is the exception of course). They are depressing and as the journey toward survival ensues, they will only further confuse you and distract you from relaxing. I'm really lucky that I found the lump by doing self-breast exams (or having fun in the shower—however you want to look at it). Most women with this type of cancer don't go in for help before it has penetrated every organ—okay, I'm exaggerating, but that's what it seems like. One blog I was reading made the whole experience sound like a death sentence. Luckily, for the most part, I stick to the scientific journals where at least I can keep some emotional distance from the subject.

However, the results are mixed on outcomes and a lot of the participants are older women in their 50s and 60s. So I find more comfort reading the journal articles looking for flawed methods and low numbers of participants. For example, if you read a study where six people were followed who ate fish every day for seven months and suddenly developed gills—six people is not a good representation of the population. Besides, my princess training (meaning I'm the ultimate princess) has taught me to see me as the exception in every case.

On the last visit to my breast cancer surgeon, she mentioned again to me that I should really be working on cutting my hair. I was like, "Are you kidding me? Didn't you notice that I already cut off four inches?" I don't think I will tackle the whole haircut thing again until I meet with the oncologists in the next week. I would like to put out a thank you to my dear friend who sent me a website of "slutty wigs" that I could try. I was kind of thinking that maybe I would try the whole Sinead O'Conner thing for a while. It might work as long as no one asks me to sing, then the gig is up. No one wants me to sing.

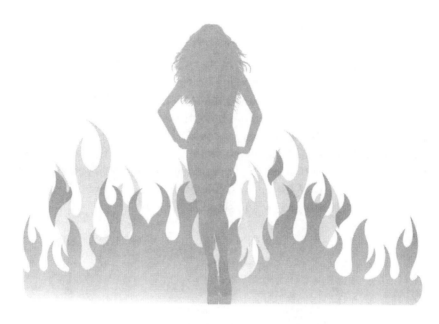

8 THE NEXT STEPS

June 8, 2010

As I suspected, this whole "I have cancer" thing has kind of hit me since the surgery. Of course, some of this might have been avoided if the damn plastic surgeon hadn't overfilled my expanders. This has caused a lot of pain, which makes me very tired. Every doctor that I have talked to about this just shakes her head, saying that plastic surgeons just don't think about the pain. Thus, my excitement for writing comes in waves.

To further compound this, my own expectations for an easy recovery were extremely overestimated. I spoke to a doctor today, and she again just shook her head when I mentioned that I wanted to get back to traveling for work. She, like so many others, have reminded me that this was a major surgery—not laparoscopic. I tell patients so often when I talk about weight loss surgery how minimally invasive it is, and I guess I convinced myself that this would be the same thing. How completely wrong of me. As my husband once again not so eloquently put it, "They cut off two big chunks of meat. You can't expect to feel that great for a while." Yes, even the psychologist has her own issues. It's hard going from 100 miles an hour to waiting for the latest episode of "Glee" to be on. Normally, I would use such down time to read a textbook or do some online CEUs. I mean, let's at least get some use out of this time. But guess what, my brainpower is less than normal. Medications for pain will do that to you.

Last Thursday, I had my appointment with my breast surgeon to go over my surgical pathology report. It was all really good news. Apparently, she got all of the tumor. I would hope so, seeing that she took both of my entire breasts! The tumor had good margins, meaning no cancer sneaking out and beyond where I feared most. The tumor was far from my skin and my chest, which reinforced that I will not need radiation. Dr. Breast Cancer Surgeon is very positive, and as a result, I will only need to see her when I get a port in my chest for chemotherapy in about three months.

That's one of the things that cracks me up about surgeons—all of them—including the ones I work with. Before the operation, everything is on fast-paced emergency mode. You really start to bond with the person, and then after the surgery, it's "See you in three months!" Just as soon as you're liking a person, they cut off the relationship. What if I grow a second head by then? I was assured by staff that I can make an appointment and get in to be seen without a problem—even if I don't get a second head.

The next happy stop was to meet with the perky oncologist at her special spa-like office. As I walked in, there was a woman well into treatment. She was bald and wearing a yarn-knit pink snowcap. In case you're wondering, I will not be wearing a pink thick-yarn snowcap.

She was a transient in cancer and we passed one another with downward glances.

It has been a couple of weeks since I met with Dr. Oncologist. When I was called back to get my vitals, I was happy to see that the student who took my vitals the last time seemed to actually know how to use the machines. I was psychically willing all of my calories to go to my breast tissue so that I would lose at least 20 pounds after surgery. Well, when I got on the scale, I didn't lose 20 pounds, but I did lose a few. One of the other medical assistants also reminded me that my breast expanders with the saline did weigh a significant amount, so I could take that into account! See the power of the mind?

■

The student medical assistant led my mom and me into a

consultation room again like last time. We go past an area with flip flops, scarves, earrings, broaches, and wigs that were all for sale. Most of the items were things that one might find in an old lady accessory shop. This seriously makes me wonder if chemotherapy somehow turns one into a tacky dresser, but the jury is out on this one. After all, when I wear a t-shirt that is not white, people wonder if something is wrong with me.

This time Dr. Perky Oncologist enters the consultation room with her physician's assistant—a guy—whom she doesn't introduce. I'm thinking that I'm not taking my top off for this guy, especially with no introduction. Anyway, Dr. Oncologist has my surgical pathology report and is a notch below the usual perkiness. She goes on to explain to me that the tumor is 75% metaplastic tumor and 25% of the tumor looks like a "regular" type breast cancer. The estrogen receptors and HER2 are both negative, but the progesterone is still slightly positive—which is not normal either. This is quite the dilemma for her—which is not a good thing in my opinion when a doctor is in a dilemma about a tumor. She mentions that she is going to present my case to the tumor board at the local hospital and will send slides to the experts at UCLA.

Apparently the dilemma is that the tumor represents less than one percent of all breast tumors. It's usually seen in much older woman and is more common in African American woman. And here I was, complaining the first couple of months of the year about turning 40 this year. Now, all I'm hearing from doctors is that choosing my treatment is complicated by *how young I am*. Go figure.

Dr. Oncologist proceeds to tell me that her initial treatment plan is to start me on chemotherapy on June 21, 2010 with a higher level of A/C treatment every two weeks for four cycles—this is instead of the every three week treatment she talked about initially. As an added bonus, after the day of the chemo, I get to come back and get some shots to make sure I keep up my white count with scheduled follow-ups. I mentioned to Dr. Oncologist that, "Gee, that schedule kind of puts a damper on the whole traveling thing between treatments that you mentioned before." To her credit, she did say that traveling is possible, but basically with that much chemo happening so close together, I probably won't have the strength to pull my own overhead luggage bag. But if I do decide to travel, I can "always call her." I'm obviously not going anywhere.

This more aggressive treatment she is going for could get worse depending on the tumor board and what she gets back from the experts. Again, I ask, "Now let me get this straight. After all this, we'll not be able to tell if the chemo is working?"

Yep—again... that's how insurance works, but once again, because of my "youthful age", chemo is recommended. Since this type of cancer generally metastases to the chest and lungs, not the lymph nodes— chest X-rays every three months may be a part of my routine for a long time. I'm glad that Dr. Oncologist is perky like I am or else we might have a problem.

So, the next step?

Dr. Oncologist and her staff will call me to set-up a "pre-chemo class" and a heart test since the medication can wreak havoc on your heart. I hope that the "pre-chemo" class does not include how to wear tacky scarves. I'm really hoping for more on how I can sneak a glass of wine in between treatments. Oh, and finally, I have to set-up another operation to get the port in so that the medications and blood draws can be done "oh so conveniently" without wearing out my veins.

I restrained myself from asking if I had a choice between a port that looked like Sponge Bob or Brad Pitt—pre-Angelina. Again, I tried to find out if there was a type of chemo I could take that could stop me from losing my hair—but no luck on that one. I will be overdosed on anti-nausea medication so it won't be like "the movies" as she put it.

It finally hit me that the pathology report was not wrong, and the emotional swaying that ensued made me come ever so closer to the reality of my condition without all of the comedy I had tried to clutter into my mind. I have cancer. It's a rare cancer. It doesn't have much literature or clinical trials to go by. I'm me, but my cancer was something else.

Several separate pathologists have looked at the slides and are coming up with the same reports. My lottery analogy was fading, and the dream of a medical mistake faded. If I have a type of breast cancer that is less than one percent of all breast cancers, my luck with the lottery has to improve.

The question of my hair also starts to creep into my mind, especially as my mother kept asking me constantly. All through this, my mother is walking around with a boot because of her broken ankle. Getting out of the car together with her limping and me walking like an 80-year-old woman, we are something to see. But we both remain women, mothers, and warriors.

■

On Saturday, I looked up wig shops. Have you ever been to a wig shop? I mean for something other than an Elvira wig for Halloween. Well, in case you didn't know, Raquel Welch has quite the corner on the market for wigs and they are damn expensive. My mom and I walk into the wig shop and of course, there is a woman who is about 110 working the counter—well, actually 71 years old—she told us. I really had to behave myself because there were SO many comments that I could have made. My mom kept looking at me like, "Don't you dare say anything." I completely expected to cry through the whole thing, but I didn't. It was not that bad. 71-year-old lady was actually was very helpful and really knew what she was doing. She said, like everyone else, that it's a good thing that I came in before I lost my hair so I can match a wig more closely to my own hair. I have to say that I was shocked at how nice some of them were. Not only that, but I can bring the wig back and have it trimmed if necessary. Again, I know I'm adorable, but even in a wig—who knew?

She had a long Elvira one but that one made me look like a cheap hooker—so that one was out. After trying on several, I settled on one and actually walked out with a wig. Of course, I haven't had it out of the bag since I bought it. Denial is a damn strong emotion. After looking around the shop, I can totally see that there are probably a lot of people who wear wigs—and I don't mean Lady Gaga—and none of us know it. Again, the hope is I'm that one percent of chemo patients that do not lose their hair. I mean if I have a type of cancer that only one percent of people get...you never know.

I was feeling pretty good that day about the whole thing. I told my mom that I thought we would have lunch and then do some shopping. Another ambitious moment on my part. I made it through lunch, barely. It was back to nap time at the Ponderosa.

Since I overdid it that day, I was in bed more of the next day. Being pissed off about it, with the weakness and fatigue slowly laying their claim upon me. I think I have written all I can tonight before the Vicodin kicks in.

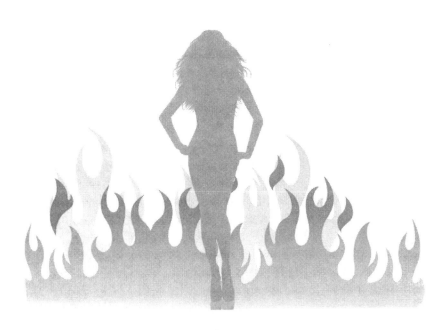

9 DEBBIE DOWNER TIME

June 14-17, 2010

Denial is getting the better part of me. The last week has been particularly tough after I went to another Cancer Center for a second opinion. The physician was great, but was not what I would call touchy-feely, but Dr. No Bedside Manner. She really laid out the statistics, stating there are no good studies for metaplastic cancer and its response to chemotherapy. Instead, any chemotherapy I get will target the 25% of the tumor that is more of a "regular" type cancer. Then she ended her talk with me on the note that if the metaplastic metastasizes to the bones or lung, it will be basically incurable. She actually said, "You'll be toast." Who says that to a patient?

Walking out of that discussion didn't leave me as the usual positive person that I am. Yet between this and the recovery from the surgery, it has really knocked the wind out of my sails. I'm waiting to have an appointment with my local perky oncologist to get out of this slump. I did talk to my breast surgeon who'd put in my chemo port, an attractive accessory to my chest. She basically told me that she hand-picked a superior team to help with my cancer. I needed to trust her. I should have talked to her first before getting the second opinion. Apparently she knew about Dr. No Bedside Manner.

On the bright side, I did discover one of the benefits of having expanding breasts versus real breasts. When I went to the grocery store and was in the refrigerator section, I didn't have to worry about nipples showing—because I have none! I know...too much information, but I have to find the benefits where I can!

The other thing I think I forgot to mention was that I had to get a bleeding test before my mastectomy to make sure I wasn't a super bleeder on the table. When I had my kids, I had to be given massive amounts of medications to stop the bleeding. When I finally found a lab that would do the test, I had to sign all of the usual consents and one line mentioned that I might get a small scar. I didn't think too much about it until the lab tech mentioned it by saying, "You know you're going to have a scar, right?" The device they use to make the prick in the skin to make it bleed is probably no bigger than the tip of a pen. I started laughing and told the tech that was the least of my worries— seeing that after my surgery I would have massive scars across my chest. I don't think one tiny scar on my arm is going to be a big deal.

■

I'm really trying to keep my attitude up about all of this for a number of reasons. As you have probably read, studies in which people who have a positive mental attitude heal faster and are able to combat illness easier. But you know what? That's easier said than done.

In very exciting news, I was in an upright position (meaning not laying down) for almost a whole five hours today. I think I might actually be healing from the surgery.

Dr. Perky Oncologist found out from her staff that I was a mess and actually called me herself yesterday (or was it today?)—these days all run into each other. I told her the situation that I felt that I should at least get another opinion about chemotherapy and treatment before things get started just, for peace of mind. She was wonderful about it. I told her about who I saw at the other Cancer Center, and Dr. Perky immediately said, "I know her. We compete for the same articles and on the lecture circuits within the oncology community." There is a reason why people are in academic institutions and can't make it in private practice. They have no people skills. Dr. Perky was definitely successful with her private practice.

She told me not to worry and that this particular doctor does not have a way with patients. Dr. Perky mentioned that she has already sent my tumor slides off to both a local and an international tumor board to try to figure out why I have negative estrogen, but slightly positive progesterone receptors—which is apparently rare.

She is also considering adding a medication to the chemotherapy cocktail that targets lung cancer, since that's usually where the metaplastic cancer goes first—there and the bones. She was very positive about it. I'm scheduled on Thursday for some type of test to make sure my heart can handle all of the chemo they are going to give me. So, tentatively the start date of chemo is June 21, 2010, but now with all of the experts Dr. Perky is consulting, this might be postponed— which is fine with me. Dr. Perky usually doesn't like to start chemo until five weeks after the mastectomy, just to make sure everything is healed before my immune system is hit by a truck. June 21st would only be slightly more than four weeks.

Since I was feeling better today, I actually left the house. I went and got my haircut a little shorter—and yes, I went back to Not-So-Normal Girl. She was really sweet. I brought the wig in with me because it has kind of long bangs and I have never had bangs in my life. She seemed to do a good job but you know how haircuts are—you never know how they are until you work on it yourself. So far, I have enough hair to still poof it up on those fat days. However, I will say that having a mastectomy with just little mounds where the expanders are does seem to shave off the pounds. Of course, my V-neck white tee (because you know that is all I wear) where I show cleavage is out—unless I want everyone to see my surgical old lady bra and port site. If you think about it, sometimes it's quite sexy to see a little bra strap here and there... but not if you got a look at this bra I'm wearing. I really can't even tell if it's doing anything or not, just that I've been told to wear it at all times. Lucky me.

Another positive thing happened. My son's old teacher hooked me up with a mother in his class who's also had cancer; apparently much worse than mine. She sent me a very inspiring email and gave me some great suggestions for vitamins and minerals to help with my immune system and energy. I'm forever thankful for that. So, after I got my haircut which is nothing near short, I went next door to the local health food and vitamin shop. I have to admit that I played the cancer card. I showed the sales lady the email with the nutrition stuff on it and she knew exactly what it was, and they had it in stock. I got a little teary-eyed and she was just great. Apparently she lost her grandmother to breast cancer. So now I have a load of supplements that I will have to check out with my doctors to make sure I can take them. I'm sure most of them are benign, but you never know. Believe it or not, that little bit of teary-eyed-ness at the nutrition shop and having Not-So-Normal Girl cut my hair was the only real crying I did today. I think that is quite an improvement.

However, controlling the crying on the phone is a little harder. I think that Dr. Perky got me back on track, and my attitude is a little better. So I'm not avoiding anyone. I just can't always get my shit together to talk about all of this. I appreciate all of the cards, flowers, and cookies (chocolate is always good). Of course, I can't help but think that my house is beginning to look like a funeral home. But that's probably because I have never been a domestic goddess and have probably never, and I mean never, bought even a bouquet of flowers for my house. You know, like people go to Trader Joe's and buy these lovely flowers—I guarantee you have never seen me walk out with one of those. If you did it, was mistaken identity. I usually go for the plastic ones that are harder to kill.

Another thing I have to admit is that because I have no energy and am not as hyper as usual, I haven't been able to spend a lot of quality time with my kids. Not that they seem to care. They have their own rooms now, and a pool. My son hardly wants to leave the house. Early last week when I was in real Debbie Downer mode, I did hit Toys"R"Us and bought them some toys they didn't need. Of course, they loved them—for about the usual five minutes—before they wanted something different. So the kids seem fine and unaffected by all of my own drama. Being a psychologist doesn't always work at home.

When you have cancer, the priorities change. Things like little projects that my husband can't seem to get done, or cleaning out the garage, don't seem to bother me. My own office at the house is completely cluttered with books, reports and, of course, I have a cancer section now. Even crap left on the counter in the kitchen that used to drive me half mad doesn't seem to matter as much. I mean if the president and the first lady were coming to dinner, I would probably tidy up a bit but other than that, eh, not so much.

When people call me on my phone and I don't recognize the number and am not in the mood to talk, I don't answer. It's truly amazing how one phone call can change your entire perspective on life. Before the call from my primary care doctor on May 4th telling me I had cancer, I was worried that my key to my new mail box wouldn't work. That doesn't matter now. But what the hell am I going to do for eyebrows once my hair falls out? That seems to be a much bigger deal at this moment! Since I'm blonde I have never had to worry about "shaping" my eyebrows, because you can hardly see them anyway.

If we get a chance to go to Disneyland during this whole thing, you can damn well bet that I'm using the cancer card and getting a wheelchair to get on the rides first! Not sure if I will be able to go, but I definitely will have that planned out! Heck, I've seen families pushing around Grandpa who's got almost both feet in the grave, just so they can get on *It's a Small World* before everyone else.

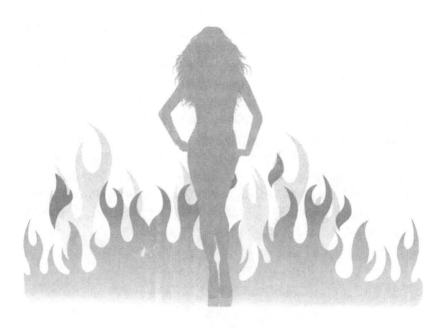

10 CANCER SUCKS

June 21, 2010

I feel more like a human being than I have in a long time. Tomorrow will make it four whole weeks since my surgery. I still get tired very easily but I feel like I can at least walk up the stairs. Today I had something called a MUGA (I think that's the way it's spelled) scan. They take your blood out and put it with some radioactive isotope, then put it back in. The nurse used my new handy port that was installed last week. It was actually kind of cool—except for the part where she missed it the first time. Yeah, that felt good. Then they take about 100 pictures as a baseline to see what my heart looks like. And why do they do that, you might ask? To see just how much damage the chemotherapy will do to my heart. Nice. At least I got a blanket to keep me warm during the process.

After that fun appointment, I got to go back and see my buddy the plastic surgeon. Since my expanders were hurting so much the last two times, he didn't fill them. This time I got them filled up with more saline. If you see me around, don't accidentally bump into me in the chest. It's not me I'm worried about; you might get injured. It's like I have two rocks on my chest. At least if I fall in the pool, I won't drown. I come with my own floatation devices to bring me back to the surface. That's what recovery is after all, right? After going through this, I really don't understand why anyone would want to voluntarily get breast augmentation. This must be why celebrities stay in hiding before "coming out"—they're in bed and in pain.

As far as my chemotherapy start date—I'm not really sure. I was tentatively told Monday, June 21st, but I haven't gotten the call to receive the "pre-chemo" class. However, I kind of figure that the oncologist office assumes that those of us with cancer kind of keep our schedule open. If they call tomorrow and tell me to start tomorrow, I will show up at whatever time they tell me.

I've been thinking about some of the tidbits that come with having cancer. For example, I'm almost out of my Blonde Expression shampoo. What to do, knowing that my hair is going to fall out soon? Do I spend the money on it and have shampoo that I can't use in my shower for months? I figured I could buy some since my daughter's hair is blonde, we can use it on her. Do you realize how big the section in Target is for hair products? There are at least four aisles dedicated to shampoo, hair spray, dyes, curlers, etc. I guess I'll be saving money on that for a while. Of course, my husband has been wanting to shave his head for years now, so he's volunteered to shave his head when I have to shave mine. I'm sure it's a gesture of love, right?

Another issue that seems to come up is the "who do you tell?" situation. When I got my haircut again, I did tell Not-So-Normal Girl and she was very sweet. I mentioned it to the woman I purchased some vitamins from—thus the reason why I'm buying vitamins—and she tells me her long, sad story of losing her grandmother to cancer. I didn't really need that pep talk.

Most people are pretty compassionate and appropriate. However, I keep thinking about this couple I saw in therapy years ago. They were in their 60s. They spent a whole session talking about how their friend got cancer and had chemotherapy and how it was the worst thing ever. And if they ever get cancer, they won't do anything. They would rather have the cancer take them. Their combined passion about the whole thing still sticks with me.

By the way, I think that the vitamins are helping—at least on a placebo-effect level.

The most helpful people I've met are the ones who have in

confidence told me that years ago they had breast cancer and how they dealt with it. This has been most beneficial. I finally feel like I'm not a wimp because I'm still in the recovery stage of the surgery. Most women have to take six to eight weeks off. This certainly is not a club I wanted to join, but it does seem that membership comes with support. Think about it: one in eight women will be affected by breast cancer at some point in their life. Those are pretty scary odds. I think the probability is that I, and I suppose the rest of us, think that we are special somehow and are not going to be one out of the eight. Of course, I'm still taking this as a sign that I will be winning the lottery very soon. Kind of like that episode of *Seinfeld*, "Even-Steven."

The other thing I was thinking about was going through some of my clothes and other things that I probably won't be able to wear after all this. Then I thought that with all of the therapist friends I have; they would see this as a pre-suicidal sign. That is definitely not the case.

■

My oncologist told me that I would probably start chemo today—June 21, 2010. Well, I still have a pre-chemo class and some other stuff. Apparently the chemo nurse has to figure out my schedule so they will get back to me. See, this is part of what sucks. Being a doctor (well, not a real one—just a psychologist), I now know what it means to have to wait to have the damn doctor's office call you back. As a patient, it seems likes ages.

"Did they forget about me?"

"Maybe things aren't as bad as I think they are if they're taking their time getting back to me?"

Like a regular old patient, I wait. I'm not good at it, particularly now that I have no concentration or focus for any length of time. I have to work in spurts.

Another thing about cancer that sucks is the exhaustive research I have been doing. I research everything when I have questions—but when it comes to my own cancer, this can be daunting. I'm reading journals, going on NIH, looking up stuff on Medline. But you know what? I read last night that rarely do people under the age of 49 get this type of cancer.

Could my curiosity be contributing to some new depression? Or is it just the cancer?

You know what else sucks about cancer? No doctor can tell you if they got it all. Sure they got the whole tumor, the margins were clean, there was nothing in the lymph nodes. *But* there is always that small chance that one rogue cell broke away from the pack like a wild dog, imbedding itself into another place in my body and start to reproduce in its newfound haven. And hence we reach the sucky reason behind chemotherapy, annihilate the enemy, even if the doctor can't tell you if the chemo is working.

That's why I will need scans of my body for the rest of my life. Indeed, cancer sucks.

I haven't even started chemo and I'm dreading it already. I have the handy dandy port in so that my veins will be conserved and preserved.

I hear mixed reviews. Some people say that it's hell on earth. Others say, "Oh honey, it's not that bad." Being somewhat of a control freak, this unknown stuff sucks. What if my body explodes the second the medicine starts dripping into the port? What if I'm the only person on record who has her hair fall out as she gets her first chemo treatment! The mind is a wonderful thing, isn't it? It can just come up with stuff.

I had a pretty stressful weekend—again, partly my own fault for looking up stuff on the internet about metaplastic cancer and survival rates. Pretty much the literature is mixed and there is no standard method of treatment for it. So it will be interesting to see what my oncologist comes up with. I'm envisioning the green slime stuff that they splash on people at the *Nickelodeon* awards. So yes, there were tears. I do feel like I'm improving. I really think a big part of this problem for me is the fatigue. I'm constantly tired. I'm used to doing 17 things at once and I can hardly pay attention to a television program.

You know what else sucks about cancer (men, close your ears)? These damn surgical bras. I have to wear one at all times and they're ugly and come up really high. I struggle to find a white t-shirt out of my closet that will cover the bra. I have a nice sports bra that zips up the front, much like the surgical bras, but since my plastic surgeon seems destined to fill up my expanders until I'm Dolly Parton, Jr., that one doesn't fit anymore. Ugh.

I hate that it puts your life on hold in so many ways. I really can't plan a trip. I don't know if I can handle a long car ride. I read that when you have lymph nodes removed (I only had one or two removed), a plane ride can cause lymphedema. That's what I was doing every single week before this happened. You also tend to get a little over-sensitive about your body.

I didn't feel particularly well yesterday. So, right away, my mind takes control of the senses and shoots questions that I can't keep up with—has the cancer spread?! My lips are chapped. Is that a sign of something? The skin around my port is really dry—what does that mean?

I feel like I have intern's syndrome like when I was in graduate school, and we all thought we had every diagnosis in the DSM. Well, most of us had to have a little bit of obsessive compulsive disorder to get through. Also, my outings are limited. I get tired so fast that if I stay out all day, and then I get emotional. It's a vicious cycle.

The other thing cancer seems to do, and I do apologize for this ahead of time, is that it makes you somewhat selfish. I seem to be consumed with pain, what's happening with my body, are my kids happy, are they affected by this at all? It all seems to be about me lately. I'm not comfortable with that, but that's just the way it seems to go. Tomorrow I go to the plastic surgeon to get "pumped up" some more, but to be honest, I don't know how we can get that much more into those babies!

Of course, there are some things about this experience that have not been completely horrible. I have learned that life will go on if I slow down. I don't have to do 17 things at once, and the world will keep moving. I have learned that I have to rest. I learned that having over 100 channels on cable really can mean that there is nothing good on. I have found that I have wonderful, caring friends who continue to remind me of that at just the right moments of the day. My husband has really stepped up to the plate through all of this as well. He is right on it, getting me something if I need it. He is okay when I need to take a nap. He snaps me out of my depression when I feel like I'm not going to make it.

And, even better, a cute pair of shorts that I have that were tight a couple of weeks ago are loose on me now. How cool is that?

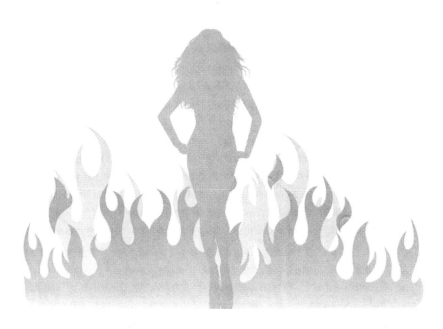

11 THE WAITING GAME

June 23-29, 2010

The receptionist called to tell me that she still wants me on the calendar with the oncologist in a month. She spoke to the chemo nurse and my chemo will be starting next Wednesday, June 30th at 9am. At that time, I will have a little mini-seminar on all of the possible side effects that come along with chemotherapy. In the meantime, she said I had to pick up two anti-nausea medications so I can start taking them before chemotherapy. This is a little worrisome. The doctors keep telling me that chemo is not going to be that bad, but apparently I will be jacked up on so many drugs I won't know the difference—or at least, this is what I'm thinking, anyway.

I have pretty good insurance coverage except for the fact that my insurance does NOT cover name-brand drugs—only generic. I was prescribed a three-pill pack of a drug called Emend. I'm thinking at most it'll be $20 a pill. Oh no, it was $344.00. YES, THAT'S RIGHT! THREE HUNDRED AND FORTY-FOUR DOLLARS! I think that I might just have to strip and pick up the spare change to pay for that. I emailed the company about getting help to pay for it. And, of course, I can get it in Canada for almost a third of the price. I guess I can't complain. I just got the EOB from the hospital visit and they charged Blue Cross $55,000! Wow. These are going to be some expensive breasts.

Now that I know my chemotherapy is going to start next Wednesday, what does one do to pass the time? I'm definitely staying off the internet research sites because then I will be clinically depressed for days, so that's not an option. I thought that maybe I should read some of the literature that the nice lady from the American Cancer Society gave to me when I was at the Arizona Cancer Center. She was the nice lady—not the doctor. I got a handout on how to battle the fatigue that comes with this whole process. It's the fatigue that's bumming me out. I'm not a sit-on-the-couch-and-read-trashy-novels kind of girl. I like to move, keep busy, and experience more beyond my living room.

Anyway, I open up this brochure on *How to Manage Fatigue*. What is the first line that jumps off the page? "Fatigue can be a sign that the cancer has come back." That was almost laughable. Just what I want to hear. Maybe my eyes were looking for it there in the mess of words, and perhaps my mind was focusing on only the bad news. But it stood there and imprinted itself in my fears.

I was also given some big books from the American Cancer Society as well as a journal from a "Live Strong" seminar with Lance Armstrong. I started to read it and the first thing it starts to describe is the difference between an inpatient facility and an outpatient facility. I'm a wee bit ahead of that. No offense, Lance.

Some of the other books I've been given have been pictorials of men and women who've lost their hair after chemotherapy doing what they do. I'm not quite ready to look at that book yet, either. Although I will, but definitely not today. I'm still working on disassociating myself or detaching myself from my hair. I got it cut a little shorter with some wispy bangs—which I've never had in my life—I'm still getting used to it. The easiest way to deal with this is to have my hair pulled back. I thought about going in for another short pixie-type haircut, but since it will most likely all fall out in a matter of weeks—why try? I probably would hate that even more since I'm hardly the "pixie" type of girl.

I will say that my husband has been supportive and said that he and my son will both shave their heads once my hair goes. As I can't get near my daughter with a brush, I doubt shaving her head is an option.

Other things to pass the time while waiting for chemotherapy....I could read some of my scholarly journals and other books, but the problem is that the Valium I'm on for my expanders makes it hard to concentrate on *People* magazine, let alone anything scholarly. Speaking of that, I went to the plastic surgeon yesterday for my final "fill-up" of my expanders.

The idea of the expanders is to expand the muscle and the skin for the new implants. However, the expanders have expanded slightly to the side. I mentioned to Dr. Plastic Surgeon that I'm not interested in having side boobies. He assured me that this will all be fixed when I have the next surgery. I don't have to go back to see him for another three weeks. I don't know how much more these expanders could handle, although my husband argued that they could probably handle a lot more. I was talking to the receptionist and asked her about how people do this to themselves with breast augmentation. She said that most of those patients say it's hell for about a week after surgery. At this point, I really cannot imagine doing this to myself on purpose.

But, you never know. I also saw a 70-year-old woman in the lobby of the plastic surgeon's office getting Botox. I might change my mind when I'm 70.

I think the worst part of waiting is having all the thoughts come back to your head from everyone in the world who has told you in the past how horrible chemotherapy is. I had a patient tell me about her daughter. She said one time the chemo nurse administered the first round of chemo too fast, and she started to have a seizure. Yeah. Happy thoughts.

Or I have these fantasies that I'll be the one patient whose hair falls out completely by the end of the first chemo session. I might be forced to purchase one of the scary scarves on display at the doctor's office before I leave. Or what if I turn purple or green from the drugs? Those are not good colors on me. Royal blue would be better.

I had one person tell me that the surgery is the easy part; it's the chemo that's worse. How is it that I meet only the "motivational speakers" on this subject?

Since I've had to significantly cut back on work, as cancer tends to interrupt that as well, I don't want to go spending a lot of money, either. Conversely, I can't work myself to death on projects that I have had on hold until I have had the time. I get worn out. I have a short window of time where I have clarity enough to work and get things done that require mind power. I anticipate that this will lessen as chemo progresses. I think I mentioned before that I went to the bookstore trying to find some inspirational books on cancer, and the book I picked up is called *Chemo Brain*. This book outlines how some people on chemo have a significant cognitive decline and for some, it never comes back! I quickly put the book back and went to a different section of the bookstore. Fabulous.

So, in the meantime, I think I'm going to take the approach that a wonderful friend has told me...relax...watch funny movies and television, etc. And guess what? There are actually studies that indicate that people who do that increase their immune system functioning. Finally, a study that doesn't scare the shit out of me. Of course this will be a bit of a battle, since I do have leisure time activities issues. I have none.

■

Wednesday is fast approaching. My mother arrives on Tuesday. I just got the treatment protocol via email from the oncologist's nurse. Have you ever read the inserts of the medications that you've been prescribed? Yeah. Most of us don't. But it's hard not to when there are over SIX pages of possible side effects of the medications that will be pumped through my veins. Oh, and I also got a handout on managing nausea. Real excited about that one. Those $300 pills better take care of that or I will be back at Walgreens beating the pharmacist for my money back. To be honest, I just scanned the side effects because I didn't want to depress myself. I have done enough of that lately.

I have to say that I'm SO tempted to Google "worst case scenario chemotherapy treatments." But, why? It's like looking at a car accident or a train wreck. For some reason, we just can't look away. You'll be happy to know that as of this writing, I have not done any such Googling.

A friend and her daughter came over today and it was a wonderful distraction—not just because they visited, but because they're wonderful people. My best friend in Illinois hooked us up. We both barely know anyone here, so it's a nice match. Of course, my son has already told her daughter that he "loves her" and that she is "hot". He's seven. I don't know where he gets this stuff. We're working on boundaries with him, or else the entire park would be at our house every time we went.

I do feel like I'm more or less recovered from the surgery. I'm still low energy and the rocks on my chest are really annoying, but I'm starting to think more clearly and my body doesn't feel like it has been hit by a truck. Of course, I have Wednesday to look forward to. At that point, all of this might change.

I was reading some of the side effects of chemotherapy and, of course, one of them is hair loss. I had to laugh. It recommended that you not "perm or color" your hair and that usually chunks of hair will fall out on your pillow and while showering. Now why in the world am I going to perm or color my hair when I know it's going to fall out? Bell curve. I have to keep reminding myself that there are many people on the far left side of the bell curve who might find that information useful (a little psychologist humor). Of course, there are many things that I haven't read that I probably should before Wednesday, but instead I think I will just say a little prayer and leave it in God's hands.

■

My chemotherapy starts tomorrow at 9am. I just called up the chemotherapy place and asked the kid at the front desk to reassure me that I would not turn purple. He assured me I wouldn't. I called my aunt who just finished with chemo for breast cancer this last year. She also assured me that I would not turn purple. She did, however, tell me how she, too, thought that she was going to be the only one to have chemo and not lose her hair. To her amazement, her hair did start to fall out at day 10 after her first chemotherapy. And as I have heard from her and others, that part is the worst.

We have a wonderful woman who helps me keep up the house. She sent me an email with a link about all of the famous bald women in the world. Of course, the first one was Britney Spears. I think she meant to prove the point by the other ones on the list. But, it was a nice gesture. Maybe I can start a new trend. The only problem with the female bald trend versus men bald trend is that when a man shaves his head, we all kind of assume it's because he is balding anyway, and he just doesn't want the shining dome with hair around the edges.

When you see a bald woman at the store, most of us assume that she has cancer and didn't chose baldness, but you never know. Think of the conveniences—I'll be saving money on hair products. One article I read said to throw out all of the hair products in your house. Now that just seems silly. The other people in my house are still going to have hair. I read another article that even though you don't have hair, you should use a product call *Neutrogena T-gel* at least twice a week. How many of you only wash certain parts of your body twice a week? Maybe those in prison, but I usually wash up every day, as unexciting as it might be.

And for those of you wondering, given my slightly perky tone, yes, I'm scared shitless of what will happen tomorrow. Will the nurse miss the port (which happened already during another test and didn't feel very good)? Will they start hanging the bags of medicine and stop and say to one another, "Are you sure these are the right ones?" Will I be the only person who they have ever had that is immune to anti-nausea medicine? Will my head explode? Will all of my veins turn green like the Incredible Hulk?

Beside the scary stuff, there is the practical stuff to worry about. Given that that the chemotherapy place I'm going to is very "spa-like", what does one wear to chemo? The handouts I read said to wear comfortable clothes—of course, some of the women I saw were wearing designer sweat suits. Of course, I will have to pick out an appropriate white t-shirt from my vast selection in the closet. I'm having trouble finding some that cover the lovely surgical bra that I have been instructed to wear at all times. What about makeup? I'm thinking that I should at least go buy some new waterproof mascara so that if I'm crying the whole time, I'll still look halfway cute. My mom is flying in so that she can be my tagalong nurse to make sure everything goes okay for this first chemo. Are your chemo companions required to wear something that signals that they are NOT having chemo? I suppose in later sessions it's easy to figure out because they are the ones with the hair. Maybe I should make my mom wear scrubs so that she looks like she is my private nurse! She will love that.

Also, is there chemo etiquette? Most of the chemo chairs are lined up near each other so it does look like if you wanted to talk to the person next to you, you could. But that is an odd one, "Hey, you here getting chemo, too?" Do people wear their iPod ear buds in even if they aren't listening to anything because they don't want to talk—kind of like on airplanes? Will there be that one annoying chemo patient who talks incessantly—you know what I mean—there's always an annoying one in the bunch. I hope it's not me.

And what am I going to do for five hours having to sit still with IVs hooked up to me? I can't remember the last time that I had to sit still for that long—and next to my mother—no offense to my mother, of course—but five hours with anyone is a long time. If I'm going to read something—what does one read during chemo? I think it might be in bad taste to bring one of the books a friend gave me of all bald-headed women. From what I understand, they dope you up with a bunch of stuff first, so I'll probably be happy watching *SpongeBob SquarePants* for five hours straight. That's what I tell my husband, who's about nine years older than me. When his dementia sets in, I'm going to pick one DVD and tell him that it's a brand new one that he hasn't seen yet.

As I've said before, I think the fatigue is what's going to kick my ass. It has been several weeks since my surgery and I feel pretty good—except for the rocks on my chest. But I do feel like I'm getting my energy back, only to have it sucked out of me tomorrow. My understanding is that people work during the off week of chemo, but the cumulative effect of the chemo makes you really tired. I hate being tired.

Before all of this happened, I was complaining to my friends that this getting older stuff sucks because I feel tired. I want the energy I had when I was a hyperactive 12-year-old, minus the junior high drama. I started taking some supplements that someone recommended for me, and they seem to help, but then of course my mind starts to think that the chemo drugs will kill all effectiveness of even the vitamins I take.

Isn't the mind a great thing? It can take you so many places without moving a muscle. I'm going to spend the next 24 hours trying to get my mind to focus on positive, hopeful things. Again, the psychologist in me knows that people who exhibit a positive attitude do better in illness situations. I'm going to try, but there are no guarantees. Sometimes I can't get my own psychological voodoo magic to work on myself.

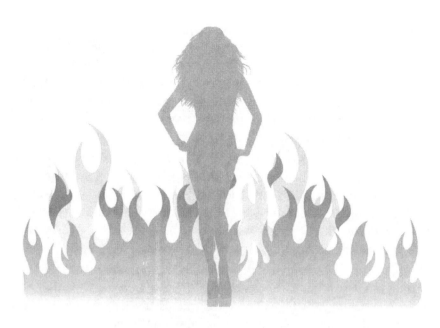

12 THE CHEMO EXPERIENCE

July 6-8, 2010

It's been almost a week since I had my first chemotherapy experience on Wednesday, June 30th. I got there early so I could have my vitals taken. As soon as I walked in, it was as if the receptionist was expecting me. It's nice when someone is waiting to receive you for dinner reservations, but not for chemotherapy. I was whisked away by the medical assistant in training, who appears to be increasing in confidence. She didn't hesitate as she did before to take my blood pressure, temperature, or pulse.

The oncologist happened to be on vacation—until the middle of July—so the oncology nurse, Michele, was my caretaker for the day. Since it was still so early in the day, I had my pick of La-Z-Boy recliners to choose from. In case I was not feeling like my witty self, which I wasn't, I chose a chair at the end that didn't have anyone on one side. This way my mom could be sitting near me in case I had to pass out or something.

When I finally sat down, my nurse was really nice and went through the whole procedure with me for the day. Thanks to my handy dandy port, all medications and saline would be put through there. I would first get a good dose of saline, then the Cytoxan. The first medication administered was the easy one.

For the next medication, the nurse actually has to sit next to me for 20 minutes and inject it into the line because they don't have the needle injection equipment or something like that. This is the "A" part of the medicine. My whole treatment is called TAC. The thing about the "A" part is that it's very red and toxic. And yes, it will be injected right into my body. The thrill, the excitement. Then the nurse put on what looked like industrial strength gloves, laid out what amounted to a puppy pee pad so that none of it would get on the furniture—but yet I get it injected in my body. I'm sure you can imagine the excitement on my face.

While oncology nurse is injecting this into me, she tells me some of the possible side effects. My pee might be look blood-red for a while. It makes you wonder about the guy who created the medications. He must have been thinking, "How toxic can I make this stuff without completely killing all of the healthy cells?"

While I'm being injected with the red toxin—which maybe I should look at in a different light—my superpower drink—the La-Z-Boy chairs were starting to fill up. Remember how I mentioned that I was worried that I would have to dress up for chemo? I was way wrong. Most of the group was not dressed up. There were people there of all ages, but of course, I have to admit I was the cutest and the youngest. Each one of the La-Z-Boy chairs has a little portable television. Of course, the chair I picked didn't because some lady stood up when she was having an allergic reaction to one of the medications and the whole thing came tumbling down. Mental note—don't stand up if I feel dizzy.

Anyway, some old guy at the other end, who seemed to be a pro, was telling people that their televisions were too loud, and he was bossing around the staff. I think being rude and loud comes with being old, but my data has not completely been calculated on that one. Another lady brought what looked like the biggest sandwich I have ever seen in my life. I didn't even think about bringing something to eat since I didn't think I would be there all day! However, surprisingly, I haven't been that hungry, so I'm seeing that as a good thing.

I was able to avoid a chair companion sitting next to me for most of the day until Nina (names have been changed to protect the innocent who have no idea I'm writing about them) came to sit next to me. Well, she did dress up for chemo, but she was not there for chemo. Apparently, if you feel weak and drained, you can come in anytime and get a bag of saline. The nurse secretly told me that no one needs as much hydration as Nina does. She, too, had the port, so I was feeling quite in style. She was walking around the center "shopping" the scarves, flip-flops, and other accessories. This is the part where I put my iPod ear buds in because I knew her life story was coming at some point.

She was a very attractive woman (as most women are where I live by cosmetic and chemical means). She seemed to have an incredible amount of energy for someone on chemo. At one point, as the nurse was pushing saline before my next drug (yes, I did it), I took my earbuds out. So, the life story of Nina is that she actually has very bad cancer and is scheduled for 18 sessions of chemotherapy.

However, when she comes, she brings her entourage and orders in food—thus, the group that I saw the first time that I visited the Cancer Center. She noted that I was sitting in her usual chair so that when she does have chemo her entourage takes up all of the empty space to the side of it. I also found out that she is a makeup artist, her daughter is a "producer", and her son is an "actor". She asked what my husband and I did—big mistake. I told her I was a psychologist which, of course, is not interesting when your husband does film finance and your entire family is trying to "get in the business." I got to see pictures of all of her kids and got her business card. At first I was like, "whatever", then I started to think that once I have no hair, eyelashes, or eyebrows; her card might come in handy. Thank goodness the oncology nurse came back to administer my next and last set of medication. Of course, my mother pointed out how chipper she seemed despite the fact she was on chemotherapy.

With this medication, Taxol—or the generic version of it, she sits down and tells me that lots of time people have allergic reactions to it. Apparently this is a very toxic medication (not that the others weren't, but this one is worse). I'm being given this one because my particular type of cancer—if it spreads—would go to the lungs and this medication would help with that. She also noted that sometimes people have allergic reactions to it, so I have to be watched very carefully. Again, the industrial strength gloves go on. She slowly starts the drip and everything seems okay.

She tells my mom to watch to see if my face flushes because that's the first thing to happen. I imagine this is a pretty easy tell since I'm about as white as you can get. In just a couple of minutes, my face starts to flush, I have shortness of breath, and as a bonus, my throat starts to close. Yeah, that really felt good. My mom waves down the nurse and the nurse yells to the physician's assistant, "We've got a reaction over here!"

Now remember, when you get chemo, you're not in a private room. I'm in a line of about 10 La-Z-Boy chairs, so now everyone knows that I'm losing it. The nurse turns off the drip and starts to give me a cocktail of drugs to stop the reaction—and wouldn't you know it—one of them is good old Benadryl. Makes you want to keep a supply of that around the house. The oncologist filling in for my oncologist comes over and starts telling the nurse and PA what to do, of course, not introducing himself. I turn around and ask, "And who are you?" I knew he was the doctor, but I was trying to make a point. At least introduce yourself, I mean, he could have been the guy who cleans the floors for all I knew.

After they get the allergic reaction under control, they just slow the drip down. I thought for sure I would at least get off the hook with that one. But no, they just slowed down the drip, gave me a bunch of antihistamine drugs and kept on going. So now of course, I'm somewhat panicked that my head might explode or something. Luckily, it didn't. Since the drip took longer, I was at the Cancer Center much longer—I opened and closed the place down. I was there for over eight hours. The nurse assured me that it would not take that long next time—probably just five or more hours.

I didn't turn purple, but I will tell you that I'm glad that she told me about my urine turning red or else I would have come out of the restroom screaming.

Finally, they push more saline into your port just to make sure that you're getting enough fluids. As I'm getting that last saline drip, the nurse brought over my next appointments. Now remember, when I first met with the oncologist, she told me that I would have four treatments every other week. So I'm figuring summer will be shot with chemo, but I can handle that. Unfortunately, things have changed. I haven't had a chance to talk with her since she was on vacation, but apparently the consensus of the various tumor boards that she sent my slides off to was that I need to have the Taxol (or whatever it is—I will have to look up the real name) each time and that stuff is very toxic—too toxic to have every two weeks, so I get it every 21 days. I kind of blurred out on this one, but I think she said either six or eight cycles of that—which means the last chemo treatment would be sometime in October. Yes, as hard as I tried, I could not hold back the tears on that one. Apparently having this type of aggressive cancer and being 39 makes the treatments more aggressive. And you know, the freaky thing is that I was really feeling old at the beginning of the year. So, at my next chemo appointment, I will meet with the oncologist and go over why my treatment schedule has changed.

I left somewhat disheartened, not only because the change in regime, but because that means I will most likely be bald for my next treatment, for my 40th birthday and for a couple months after that. One piece of good news about that, remember Not-So-Normal Girl who cut my hair? Well, she and her colleague offered to come to the house to actually shave my head when it gets to be that time. Wow. I have to say, that's pretty nice.

On Thursday, the day after chemo, I felt great. I was like, "This chemo—what's the big deal?" The only thing that really bothers me is the dang breast expanders. I really think my plastic surgeon was secretly trying to overfill me—because they're killing me. Apparently, as I have now learned, the day after chemo, you usually feel pretty good because you're hopped up on steroids. It's the days that follow—days two to four or five after chemo that you feel like crap because your body is trying to get rid of all of the stuff you just pushed into it.

It's a really strange feeling—like you get this weakness, fatigue, and brain fog where you can't focus on anything for too long. Reading anything of substance is out. Basically, the only thing that seemed even a little appealing was SpongeBob, but I decided that I should do something more productive, like "meditate"—meaning stare into space until the feeling passes. Then of course, there are all of the drugs that they send you home with to counteract all of the side effects of the medications. Apparently, you're supposed to drink almost a gallon of water. Not to worry, my mother, Nurse Hatchet, was right there making sure that I was on track with it all.

■

Most of the weekend, I was about to get up, do about an hour or so worth of stuff, and then had to lay down. Then on Tuesday, I went in for a blood draw. I guess I get these every week to see how my white blood cells are doing and such. As I was in the waiting room, the receptionist had beautiful hair. So in front of everyone, I asked if she could shave it off for when I lose my hair so I could have it. She made some joke like, "Oh, it looks awful; I was just at the gym and didn't shower." The lady sitting next to me with no hair said, "Well, it looks pretty good to us."

I had a conversation with some of the women in the waiting room who obviously had been in chemo for a while because they had no hair. They were really very supportive. I felt like I was in one of my own therapy sessions because they told me "attitude is everything." Which is usually what I tell people, but for some reason this whole cancer thing has really kicked my usual positive thinking into the slump. The ladies were so sweet and told me to ask the nurses for extra liters of saline if I really felt bad, because that can really help.

On Wednesday, I had no "perky" times and really felt like crap all day. I finally called the Cancer Center and they looked at my white count and it was 1.7. In order to even have chemo for my next time, it has to be at least 4. I said, "What about that shot you gave me—when does that work?" Well, apparently they didn't tell me that it doesn't really work for about 12 days after you get it. You just get bone pain in the meantime as a bonus. Gotta love it. I called on Wednesday night and told them I felt like crap and they scheduled me to come in today. I got to sit there again for another three hours having saline, anti-nausea, and other stuff pushed into the bag. I don't feel like running a marathon, but at least I'm upright for longer periods of time.

The nurse was then worried that maybe I had a bladder infection brought on by the chemo. So, yes, I did have to pee in a cup. I was ready to do it right in front of everyone because I feel like I take my clothes off so often for doctors, what's the difference? You'll be glad to know that I did go to the rest room. Well, then the nurse comes over and gets in at eye level, in the "I have something to tell you" position. Yes, I do have a bladder infection and they found blood in my urine. I know this stuff is really exciting to you, but I have no shame about body fluids anymore. Of course, I freaked out because Dr. No Bedside Manner at the other Cancer Center said that some of the chemo they would use on me would burn out my bladder. Apparently, this was not the case. It was mild at best and I was just prescribed more medication. You should see my bathroom sink. It looks like an old lady lives there.

The other thing is that I'm apparently in the "nadir" period, where my hemoglobin and white blood cells are at their lowest, so going out into public places is not the thing to do. I asked the physician's assistant, "So, you mean that going to Walmart and licking the carts wouldn't be a good idea at this point, right?"

He laughed and said that he wouldn't recommend it.

While I was getting my liter of fluid for nearly three hours, yes, my new friend Nina was in for her chemo with her entourage. She made a point to come over and talk to me and tell me that she wants to be friends on Facebook. I hated to tell her that I don't do Facebook for a number of reasons, so I didn't. She was giving me all the good news about how sick she has been and has been in for fluids between chemos at least three times a week. Sometimes she can't be left alone because she's so sick. Mind you, she is telling me all this while wearing a "Save the Ta-Tas" t-shirt. She is quite the character. But I have to say, she's growing on me. It's nice to have someone to talk to once and a while— of course, I would rather not hear the horror stories of chemo since I barely make it to the front door without crying. But, alas, I'm getting better.

Even though I have been thoroughly hydrated, I still don't feel fabulous, but at least not like I was bed-bound like before. Apparently I'll start feeling better soon—just in time to get my next treatment. I overheard the nurse telling my mom that the type of chemo I'm getting is really rough on the body and she hates to even do the patient education on it because there is not a lot of good news about it. The thrill. The excitement. However, I'm a big believer that everything happens for a reason. I have NO idea what that might be at this point but I'm sure it will come to me. I should start feeling better by the weekend.

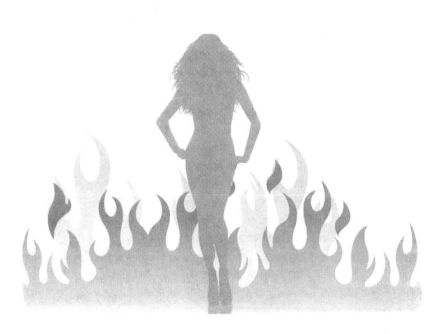

13 THE HAIR LOSS IS COMING

July 9-13, 2010

It's been 8 days since my first round of chemotherapy. The big question that I seem to ask every bald cancer patient I see: "When did you lose your hair?" Because of course, Dr. Perky told me it would be at least three or four weeks into treatment. I'm afraid I don't believe that one. I really think Dr. Perky uses the power of suggestion on me. I'm on to her. So the answers to the big hair loss question I'm getting are ranging from 12 to 15 days after the first treatment. This is no way three weeks away from the start of treatment. Any bets on when mine will fall out? Of course, you know that I'm still hoping that I'll be the one person who does not lose her hair. But if that happens, I might be slightly pissed because I've already cut off inches at the advice of my breast surgeon.

Instead of completely focusing on losing my hair like I'm sure most women do, I'm using good old psychological tricks on myself. I'm "disengaging" myself from my hair. Distancing myself from it. I've been wearing it up in a ponytail since the beginning. Making it "not a big deal" that soon I will have none. A lot of the women I've spoken to say that they wake up one morning and clumps just come out. I was thinking that on that day I might go to Target, bend down acting like I'm going to pick up something next to some unsuspecting woman, stand up, and scream that she tore out a clump of my hair. Nah, we all know I don't have the nerve to do that.

My buddy Nina at the Cancer Center told me that she fought losing her hair every step of the way. She didn't shave it until the very end. "I'm such a girl that way," she said. She went to Walmart and bought about 50 $1 bandanas and would wear those. Of course when she took them off they would be filled with hair, so she threw them in the trash when she was done with it. Not a bad idea actually. But I don't think I have "the fight" in me. I will probably go the shaving route as soon it starts. Besides, like I've said before, my husband is dying to shave his head. He's been asking me to do it since we were married, and I've always said no. Of course, now he has an excuse because he is "being supportive."

Anyway, the loss of all of my hair does really make me think about the things I value. Dr. Perky and several others have said that most cancer survivors will tell you that the hair loss is the single devastating thing of the entire process. I haven't had it happen yet so I can't put my two cents in. So far for me it has been the fatigue and the "Oh my God, I can't believe this is happening to me" feeling. I do suppose one of the advantages of going around bald as an obvious cancer patient will make using the "cancer card" much easier.

Again, I have detached myself from my hair by wearing it back in a ponytail. Nothing exciting, just a simple ponytail. All the while, I'm looking at my reflection in the mirror and saying to myself, "I'm not just my hair." "I'm not just my hair." It seems to be working, but of course I still have hair for the moment. Just keep in mind the day that I do lose my hair, my perky tone may be a notch lower than usual.

■

I got up to take a shower yesterday and, as you know, I have breast expanders. I can't have reconstructive surgery until evil chemotherapy is over, so I have these lovely stones on my chest. Well, when I went to take a shower, one of the incisions on the right side was gaping open about the size of a nickel or a quarter. I could actually see the expander! Talk about freaking out. It didn't look good. And remember, I'm in the damn nadir period where I have no white blood cells and am susceptible to infection.

Well, my husband, crossed-trained as a medic in the military, came to the rescue with the medical kit that I thought had never been opened before. He was able to put butterfly strips on it while I called the surgeon. My husband actually has a suture kit to do it himself, but I thought better of that. Knowing that the plastic surgeon is not going to send me to the emergency room and have just "some surgeon" work on his "piece of art" (that's how his office is decorated—the body is a piece of art) he prescribed antibiotics and said to keep the dressing clean. I have to go back and see him on Monday. That sucks because his office is far from my house, and I don't know how they handle this. Do they put a strip of Elmer's glue there? Use a staple gun?

The incision is obviously going to be crooked now until reconstruction—not like I'm walking around bare-chested or anything. I'm a little worried about this. Remember, this is the plastic surgeon who told me that I would most likely "just be uncomfortable" after surgery, and I then ended up staying two extra days because of pain. Maybe they have a Band-Aid in the shape of a nipple for these incidences...just like they have SpongeBob ones for little kids. Okay, that was a little off, sorry, but remember I have no nipples at the moment.

Speaking of medications, I wonder how all of those people who are "anti-medications" handle chemotherapy and this whole ordeal. I get that all the time in therapy from patients that they "don't believe in medications" as if it were a religion. I guess your tune probably changes once someone says you have cancer.

Having my mother here to help with the kids has been a lifesaver. Trying to get my kids to bed would test the patience of Mr. Rogers. Also, she's been playing Grandma with them. With me, she becomes Nurse Hatchet. "Have you been drinking your water? How much have you had today? What color is your pee? Did you take this medicine, that medicine, etc.?" Which is not a bad thing, mind you, because since I've never really been sick. I'm not good at keeping track of that kind of stuff. Before this happened, I remembered my allergy medicine, or else I would get a headache. So, I thank my mother deeply and dearly every day that she is here, and make her feel guilty every time she mentions that she is going to go home for a week or so.

Cancer can make you kind of selfish. I mean, after all, as soon as you get that call, you're on your way to doctor's appointments, surgery, therapies, and suddenly everything gets lost. Your priorities change. They kind of have to if you're going fight the battle. I've been fortunate enough to have family and friends that have come to my aide. However, I would like to single out my mom (and not just for favorite child status—I do that all the time). My mom is usually the one who is ready to help out. When my grandmother had breast cancer 20 years ago, she was right by her side. When my aunt had breast cancer just recently, she went to every chemo treatment with her.

As soon as my mom heard the news that my biopsy came back positive, all she wanted to do was to fly out and start to take care of me. The very next day, she was on a plane and flew out to my house and started to go to all of the doctor's appointments with my husband and me. She helped, I mean, continues to help, with my children. I have two children diagnosed with autism, so they can be a handful. Getting them to eat or not eat is a struggle. Getting them to listen, more difficult. However, she has been able to help with the kids and really is a supermom and ultra-super grandmom.

When we go to doctor's visits, since my head is in a cloud either due to denial or medications, she has her pink notebook and is taking notes. Oh, I have called her Nurse Hatchet a couple of times because she is constantly on me about what medications I took, did I drink enough water, am I eating. Of course, this is good because I have somewhat lost my appetite. Damn, why does it take something like cancer to do that?! When we get home, she's been making meals for all of us and then is playing Legos with my son and princesses with my daughter. All the while for part of this whole thing, I can't get off the couch.

I know a lot of people out there do not have mothers who would go to such extremes, but I'm glad that I have mine.

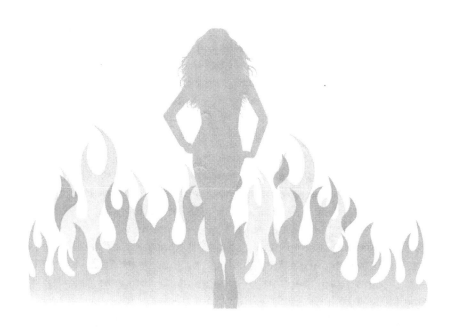

14 THE HAIR LOSS IS HERE

July 14-18, 2010

I went to shave my legs this morning and there was hardly anything to shave. I'm blonde and you can barely see that I have any leg hair if I don't shave, but I have this thing about shaving my legs every day. And today, there was no stubble. This means the hair cells that rejuvenate the fastest—which chemo kills first—are not rejuvenating. So that means that my hair is going to be gone soon. I gingerly put it up in a ponytail today, making sure not to pull too tight. The things we do to psych ourselves out, eh?

■

It's been a rather emotional morning. I got up and started to pull on my hair, and it really started to come out. I'm keeping it back in a ponytail for the next couple of days until I decide what to do. I probably don't have a couple of days, but I will try to make it last. It was really more emotional than I expected.

■

For those of you who were betting people, the hair fall-out was in the middle of the night on Friday. I woke up and felt that my ponytail holder was lower that it should be. I pulled on it and then there it was: gobs of hair came out. Then of course, in disbelief, I started to pull out more hair. I couldn't believe that it kept coming. Frankly, I was shocked I had so much hair, because I'd always considered my hair quite thin. So, I got a brush and it just kept coming. My husband was out of town, and my mom was asleep with the kids. To avoid any drama, I just worked on it myself at about 1am.

Slowly and systematically, I shaved my own head as I stared into the bathroom mirror. I scraped away whatever was left. I had desperately tried to hold onto this, hold onto what made me. And now that the time had come, I willingly submitted to the transition that cancer had forcefully brought upon me. Here I was, completely bald except for a few stubbles that seemed really stubborn. Shaving your head is not an easy task I tell you, especially the back of your head. So it looks like it took 14 days from the start of treatment to complete baldness. I'm going to have to have a talk with my oncologist at my appointment on Wednesday. She'd said at least three to four weeks, so she is going to get an earful. Luckily, I'd gone out and bought some cheap bandanas and hats the day before.

Of course, I don't think I'm leaving the house for at least six months now.

My kids are doing okay with the adjustment. My youngest really doesn't care. My mom talked to my oldest so he would be prepared. So he keeps telling me to grow my hair back by Christmas. Of course, my husband and mother have been great about it…it still doesn't mean I'm going public yet. I never realized how much hair is such an essential element of who we are. I looked online to see how cancer patients wrap the scarves and I was very scared by what I saw. I think I will be the one with the baseball cap on. Another site had women getting their entire bald head in henna tattoos. Yeah, that won't be happening, either. Of course, my loving brother suggested that I go to Walmart and go all Melissa Etheridge. My son also looks at me occasionally and says, "You're going to have to grow that hair back, you know." His innocent determination moved me.

I think the worse part of all of this is that now with no hair, it all seems very real. I mean, you'd think that with the operation and recovery period that it would be "real", but somehow losing all of your hair really makes it real. Perhaps because it's the first material thing you actually lose. Time, energy, and attitude are not things we can grasp, nor are they the first thing people notice about an individual. When I finally do go out in public, what are people going to be thinking when they look at me?

"Oh look, she must have cancer."

"Oh dear, she must be in pain."

Or worse yet, they may look away so as to not have to actualize the reality of cancer.

I did actually buy a pretty great wig, so I'll be wearing that. But when it's 111 degrees outside, that thing can get a little warm. I keep having to remind myself that this is only a "season" of my life, but it seems that it's definitely going to be one that sucks. I'm not seeing the "lesson" of all of this yet. I was happy being the autism specialist. I never had the desire to be the breast cancer specialist.

Speaking of that, I have actually opened up some of the cancer literature that I've been given since my hair fell out. Again, not really that enlightening. I mean, there's some great stuff in there about resources for support groups, financial and insurance help, etc. But when I reach the sections about the lists of symptoms to expect, the "end of life" care, I tend to close the book. I like to think I'm pretty resourceful, so I'll avoid that, and I already have the damn symptoms. I'm definitely not on the "end of life" care part yet, nor do I plan to ever reach that part due to cancer.

I plan on being like one psychologist that I read about a while ago in the *Los Angeles Times* who was still seeing patients at age 99.

I did exactly what I tell my patient to do: Take the day to do nothing and feel bad about the whole situation, then put a box around it. The next morning, realize: I have to go on with my life. Needless to say, that's what I'm doing. I'm not feeling the greatest but sometimes you just have to work through that. Being that it's a Sunday, I will take a break like the rest of the world and then get back to the pile of work I have on my desk, including getting my continuing education credits for my upcoming license.

It seems that we are given one lifetime but many opportunities to make a difference. I hope that I'm able to do that with this situation that has befallen me.

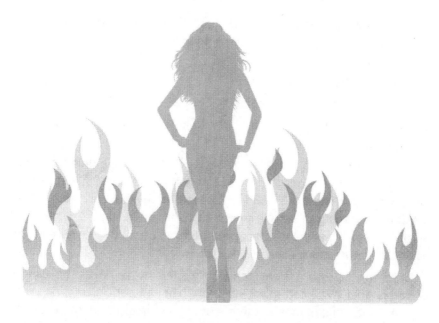

15 SECOND ROUND OF CHEMO

July 21-23, 2010

This morning, I go in for my second round of chemotherapy. I had one patient tell me it's different each time. Now that I know what to expect, I can try to use my psychological powers on myself: It will all be fine. No big deal. However, I would like to note that it's more difficult using psychological tricks on yourself. It's kind of like a surgeon stitching up a gash on his back. One might know how to do it, but it's a lot harder to do it for themselves.

As I mentioned about "chemo etiquette", I will be bringing my iPod in case any annoying patients want to tell me what their cat had for dinner. No one bothers you when you're wearing ear buds. As in every situation there is always someone loud, rude, and demanding. Also, it's a good idea to get there early and get one of the chairs on the end so you don't have someone sitting next to you. See the things I worry about now? Kind of funny since it's the same stuff you think about when you fly Southwest. What seat are you going to get? Is the person next to you going to be a talker?

In terms of things to do, I find the iPod with some books on it. I don't have the concentration to read anything too deep during day. I have an iPad, but my daughter has a death grip on it. I'm going to try to sneak it out of the house today.

I will be asking the oncologist about traveling and all of that good stuff. I'm sure she'll be oh-so-perky about it. By the way, when I went in on Monday to get my bloodwork, the receptionist recognized me even without hair. I was pretty impressed. However, having done obesity sensitivity, it makes me think that maybe they have their staff do the same thing. Something like, "Rule number one: When a new patient comes in who still has hair, focus on their face. Rule number two: Don't say things like, "Wow, I really like the shape of your head."

Speaking of that, I actually went out in public yesterday because I had to go to the post office. I know I said that I wasn't going to go, but sometimes you just have to go. I didn't get as many stares as I thought I would. I bantered back and forth with the postal worker. It took him a little bit longer to warm up than usual. Then I had to run to Target to get my anti-nausea medication for today (you know the one that I have been stripping for—the $350 for 3 pills) and everyone seemed extra-freakishly friendly. I mean, almost everyone asked if I needed any help. Not sure what to think about that. By the time I got to the register, the lady checking me out made almost no eye contact. She must not have had the "weird customer" sensitivity training. I mean, I see the people at the registers at the grocery store in town make eye contact with a cyclops and then end the conversation with a compliment.

During the last chemo, I felt great the day after because I was hopped up on steroids. We'll see how it goes this time. The thing I hate about the whole chemo thing is feeling trapped in my house. My white blood count goes so low for the first week that a kid sneezing on me in Target sets off a red alert.

In terms of my treatment goal of finding leisure skills, I hate to tell you, but it's not going very well. I did actually pick up and read a cancer brochure last night; apparently it's very common to have some forgetfulness and "chemo fog" that makes it hard to concentrate. I have been trying to read. However, I was thinking about bringing the book "How We Die" and reading that while I was doing chemo. I read it a long time ago, but to see the reactions on the people around me would be priceless. I don't think I have the nerve. Besides, they probably have some special social worker they would send over to talk to me. That might actually be fun. I digress.

I'm taking small steps. Instead of a white t-shirt, I wore a blue one yesterday; so, you never know. I might get a wild streak.

∎

On Wednesday, I was hooked up to an IV all day. And then yesterday, I had a bunch of other appointments. This chemo went pretty well. I spoke with Dr. Perky Oncologist and apparently the reason I'm on the "rough" protocol of treatment is because I'm so young and they wanted to "throw the kitchen sink at me." Great. So, I didn't have any reactions this time on the Taxol; they drugged me up ahead of time so I didn't have a reaction. And guess what? They have these steroid drugs that they could have given me last time, but they forgot. These drugs make the body aches and other symptoms go away. Nice. Well, at least I have that now. I swear I must be taking 20 pills at a time.

My mom went with me. She flies out on Tuesday to go back home (or, as I like to say, is abandoning me on Tuesday). So I will have to remember my pills and stuff on my own! Can you believe it? Well, I guess the old retiree has to go home and make sure my dad hasn't had any women in the house. In the meantime, I have met a lot of great people. As a matter of fact, the chemo nurse introduced me to a patient who just finished up her last 6th round of chemo that's similar to mine. I would like to mention that she was still bald, so I guess it takes a while to get that hair going again. I'm kind of getting used to having no hair. My "get ready" time is cut in half. No legs to shave—nothing.

Yesterday, I still felt great from all of the steroids and stuff they gave me. So we'll see how day three goes. I hope it lasts for at least a couple of days. The woman I spoke to said that she got "chemo fog" also, but that it seems to go away faster for us younger folks, which is good because I'm really catching myself forgetting things. I hate that. I hate not having any concentration. Good thing my daughter only likes me to sing the alphabet song—so at least I remember that.

During chemo, there was a woman sitting in the recliner next to me who must have been a little older than 70. She got her diagnosis of some type of cancer and since she was "so old", they didn't offer her chemo—but then the old bitty kept hanging on! So they finally decided to give her chemo and it started to help her. It just goes to show that as scary as some of the research is, you still have to read it. Her cancer went into her spine. I'm blessed that I found my lump on my own and took care of it right away, or else I might be in worse shape. So, I have those blessings going for me.

■

My mom has returned to Chicago. She actually has a life and has to get some things done over the course of August. Luckily, she stayed yesterday so I could get a liter of fluids. I've been in bed, dehydrated from my last chemo treatment that was on Wednesday of last week. I can't blame her. She's been here for over a month and then several weeks before that. I'm sure that my brother who's on the other side of the country is counting up the days that she has been here with me to make sure that he gets the same number at his house.

I'm still bald. Did you know that ALL the hair falls off from your body after chemo? All I have to do is hose myself down now when I shower. I mean, even the hair on my arms. I keep waiting to get that shallow look that chemo patients get, but it hasn't happened yet. It makes things much easier without all of that shaving. I haven't had my wig on yet because it's too hot. I had to run to the mall yesterday to pick up a new sound machine that I use when I sleep. I think people were just a little overly nice to me—which I can handle at this moment.

Yesterday, I had to go to the clinic to get my blood drawn and to get fluids. I was really dehydrated. It was super busy and almost every chair was filled up with one nurse trying to keep up with everyone. Since we all sit in a line you can get in on other people's conversations. I take Adriamycin. I overheard one nurse and a patient talking about it. They call it the "red devil" because it's so potent. Yeah. I didn't really need to know that.

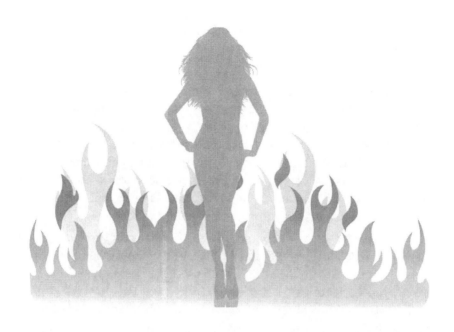

16 ADVENTURES OF CANCER WITH CHILDREN

July 29, 2010

My kids, who are seven and a five years old, have both been diagnosed with autism. The older one, my son, is actually "pretty normally developing" now. He still has problems with expressive and receptive speech, but is very social. He is probably more like a regular seven-year-old in that he talks back and gives me a hard time. The younger one, my daughter, is still in the throes of autism symptoms. Her speech has come a long way. She can say most things, but does a lot of "autistic labeling" when she communicates. For example, if you ask her something, she might say something like "Cinderella" or "Princess." However, like most kids, when she REALLY wants something, she somehow gets it out what she wants even if it's by yelling. She's progressing so we're very hopeful.

Anyway, when all of this first started, Dr. Breast Cancer Surgeon made a point for me to talk to the kids and start cutting my hair so they would not be shocked by it. I tried to explain to her that since both of my kids have autism, I'm pretty sure that my son is going to worry if he can still get Legos and my daughter won't notice or at least say anything. As I've previously mentioned, I first cut off about four inches, and then about two more. When I finally lost all of my hair, my mom talked with my son about it, and he was really sweet. She told him that I will probably grow back hair for Christmas. He saw a picture of me with hair from last Christmas and said, "That will be like mommy this Christmas." My daughter, of course, hasn't said anything. She has touched my head and still calls me "mommy", but it hasn't phased her.

As you know, my mom left. Part of her being here is helping with my daughter. My daughter is QUICK. When I say quick, I mean you cannot keep your eyes off her for more than two minutes before she gets in trouble. She's into everything. When we first moved here and had another babysitter who was more "artsy", I was ambitious and bought a bunch of paints. They went up on the very top shelf.

Well, 007, aka my daughter, has figured out that she can move things around to climb up to get them. She moved the silver trash can we have and pulled down the paints. Mind you, my husband and I had checked on her and were watching the news for literally 15 minutes. When my husband finally went to go and check on her, she had taken out about five different pieces of paper, put them on the carpet, and played Picasso. She had taken each can of paint and painted the entire page and, of course, got the corresponding color on the carpet.

Then she also decided to paint her child-sized princess table in the middle of the room. Yep, that was a fun clean-up. All of the paints went in the garbage and then I spent the next 45 minutes using our steam cleaner to get the paint out. I will still probably need to get a heavy-duty one to finish the job. Unbelievable.

Of course, she wasn't thinking, "Gee, my mom is going through chemo, this clean-up might wear her out." I'm sure that didn't cross her mind. I'm sure instead that she was wondering why her parents weren't admiring her obviously brilliant artwork.

Another issue with my daughter is going to bed. She used to be the little princess and right at 8:30pm, would lie in bed and go to sleep. No more. Now every night before she goes to bed she rocks herself to sleep either physically or vocally. Part of the routine is laying down with her and constantly redirecting her. The other problem is that she gets up at 4am and wants to play. The other night, it was my husband's turn to be on evening child patrol. The child had barricaded the door with a box of animals and said, "No, Daddy, go away." He put her back to bed. About a half an hour went by and he went back upstairs and she had barricaded the door with the mighty Wonder Pets. He said that she looked appalled that Ling Ling was not all powerful in keeping him out of the room. This went on several more times.

As you can see, chemotherapy can be exhausting, but the children really add to it. If it's not one getting into something, it's my son and his new obsession with the Titanic. He keeps building ships from Legos that are like the Titanic and then wants to spend his day in the bathtub having them sink—with the Lego people in the boat.

Obviously, I love my children and I'm happy to be home with them. However, because of my fatigue, I can't do as much stuff with them as I'd like. This doesn't seem to be a problem though, because children are creative and will find things to do on their own!

17 SICKNESS ENSUES

I was in bed a good part of the last two days because my stomach was killing me. I also thought I might have a fever. The ubiquitous feared fever of a cancer patient is never good. Most literature will tell you that you must call your doctor if you have a fever of 100.5 degrees or above. Part of the fear of this is also because my daughter has impetigo (I know, I had no real idea what it is either). It's a nasty skin rash that can really get bad. I had to bring her to the emergency room a couple of months ago because it was just scary-looking and looked like it affected her lymph nodes. So, obviously, I don't want to catch that. Our babysitter or my husband puts the cream on for me.

Thankfully, my loving mother (notice I didn't say Nurse Hatchet that time) made sure that there were thermometers strategically placed throughout the house. So, I first went to the one in the kitchen, which had not even been opened yet. It was a digital one so, having smarts but no common sense, I feared I would have to calibrate it or something. Luckily, I didn't. I read the directions, and it had a fairly simple operation. I take my temperature and, as the directions indicated it would, beeped three times if the reading was over 100 degrees. Guess what? It beeped over three times. My temperature was 101.0 degrees.

It's Thursday night about 9pm, what am I going to do? Do I call the doctor? Take a Tylenol (like I'm sure a normal person would do)?

Just to be sure about the temperature thing, I go downstairs to my bathroom and take my temperature with that thermometer. The reading is 100.5 degrees. Okay. I'm not completely panicked.

You have to understand that even though I'm a trained health psychologist, I basically know nothing about medicine. I'm trained to help you have happy thoughts about having your terminal disease or how to help you make lifestyle changes like cutting out the Krispy Kreme Donuts (which is surprisingly harder than you'd think). I also have a basic knowledge of physiology from a psychological standpoint. I actually taught a course in it. But, with real live medicine—nada. My medical expertise is calling my mother who is a nurse. My aunt is also a nurse so I have her as a back-up. I used to remember thinking, *What if something happens to my mother and I marry into a family that doesn't have a medical professional in the mix? What will I do?* Thankfully, my mother and aunt are still around.

I called my mother even though she was two time zones away—meaning about 11pm her time. She ran through my symptoms and basically went with the "take some Tylenol" route and see what happens. What would I do without her? Actually, to my credit, that was my plan as well, but being an idiot in medical issues, I needed confirmation. I took the Tylenol and eventually in the night, my fever went away.

The next morning, I didn't have a fever, but my stomach was still killing me. Part of the chemo is killing off naturally rapidly-producing cells like your hair follicles and the lining of your stomach and intestines. That's why they load you up on stomach medicine before giving you your treatment. I decided to call the Cancer Center and ask for the nurse or the PA. As I always do, I said, "Hi, it's me, your favorite patient." My theory is that if I'm chipper, I'm going to get special treatment. Anyway, I told the PA the whole fever episode and my stomach issue. He said it sounds like I have colitis. He wanted to call Dr. Perky to confirm, and would call me back. Colitis? Huh? I've heard of colitis, but I thought that's what old people got. Great. To the internet! Colitis and other intestinal issues are common side effects of the chemotherapy. And to think, I was just worried about my hair falling out.

In the meantime, before the PA calls back, I go back to bed. My kids are playing in their room. And since I have been sick, we have a great person coming in to help with cleaning and house stuff. Well, she was downstairs and so was my husband. Our babysitter doesn't get to the house on this particular day until 9am. Guess what our daughter found to entertain herself? Whiteboard markers. Her creations and manifestations were up on the walls, the wooden beams, and blinds. So I wake up from my slumber to my husband yelling that we are going to have to replace this and that. He went off to his office. I went upstairs and the housekeeper and babysitter already got most of it out. I just discovered the green marker on the blinds. We got everything off and fixed. By the way, Old English is a fabulous product. Of course, our daughter doesn't really know that what she did was wrong, so she's happy to show off her works of art. This took most of the morning.

The PA from Dr. Perky's office finally called back. By this time, I'm completely exhausted. He tells me that Dr. Perky thinks I have colitis and we need to watch the fever. So of course, this means a new and exciting antibiotic. Thank God it was generic—my insurance doesn't pay for brand name drugs if you recall. You can really get a lot of pills for $4.00 these days. I have to say the new antibiotic seems to be helping. The other great thing about being on antibiotics is it really clears your skin up. Also, now that I have so much of it showing, being bald and all, that is really a bonus.

Afterward, I laid down for my usual afternoon nap. It used to be the "why is this happening to me?" nap before the surgery, but now it seems that a little nap really helps so that I can actually do something in the evening with the kids if needed. Since I wasn't feeling very well all day, I just hosed down. Taking a shower has a new meaning. Nothing to shave, nothing to lather, nothing to condition. It really cuts down the shower time. I also didn't put on any makeup. Now I'm a pretty pale person to begin with; my legs basically glow they're so white.

After I wake up from my nap, I pass the mirror and—Oh My God!—looking back at me is a person who totally looks like a cancer victim.

No hair, and I'm about as white as one can be.

My port on my chest is visible.

Fatigue is etched around my face.

But it was still the same eyes that looked back.

I literally look like I could be the poster child for "Jerry's Kids who grew up and got cancer."

I call my best friend in Illinois to get all my thoughts off my chest- literally. Her husband answers, and guess what? She went to Paris—on her own—by herself—with no one else. She didn't even tell me. She had been trying to convince me and her other friends to go with her for a while. I can't believe she went. Of course, her husband and I discuss that top story which obviously trumped my story, which is a daily occurrence. I will have to grill her when she gets back. Of course, I'm a bit jealous since I can barely leave the house lest some toddler at Target sneezes on me.

So alas, I'm feeling better for the moment, but constrained to the house and Target (I actually go, but I'm the freaky bald white person carrying around hand sanitizer).

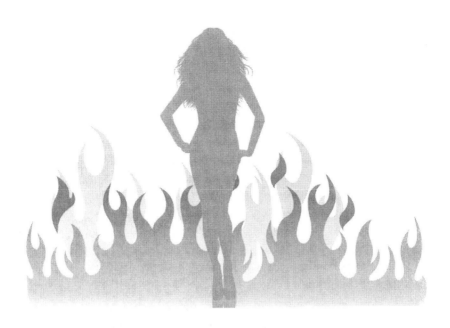

18 MISSING EVERYDAY LIFE

Yesterday was one of those "why is this happening to me?" days. I get those once in a while and I hear that I'm allowed to have them. But I don't like to write on those days because I don't want to sound like a Debbie Downer. I try to maintain strong faith, but sometimes the chaos of my life gets in the way. Every morning I wake up and cannot believe that I'm bald. I can now see why most people say that is the most devastating part of having cancer. I end up scrutinizing my eyelashes and eyebrows and hope that those don't fall out. I'm so fair-skinned that if I was stranded in the middle of an island, the one thing I would want is mascara. Vain, I know, but without it, I don't think you can tell that I really have eyes. It's a genetic flaw. Both my mother and grandmother have the same problem.

Although I was in my "why is this happening to me?" mode yesterday, I still have to get stuff done. I mean, I could just empty out a box of Cheerios on the floor for the kids and throw a couple of juice boxes in their room, but my parenting style is a little stricter than that. I actually once saw a family with quadruplets do that on television. Not to mention, my kids don't eat Cheerios. Anyway, I still try to manage to get what I can done work-wise on the computer with what little concentration I have. Yesterday, I got an email from a colleague at work whom I have always admired. She sent me the most encouraging and inspiring email. It was just what I needed yesterday.

Somehow this email got me thinking about what a crazy world we live in. Remember when you were a kid and you had all the free time in the world? You'd talk for hours with friends or go out with them. Of course, most of us still did that when we were single and didn't have kids or other obligations. If you ask me, being an adult is a lot of work that was not in the brochure. Bills, car payments, food shopping, being responsible. Ugh. Anyway, once we get to be an adult, those connections that we make with others are more transient. We have "friends" at work. But never really have a chance to spend time with them away from work. Yet, there is a connection. We don't have time to see them after work because we all have kids now, or have to attend to our duties as an "adult".

One of the things I have always said about my work is that I have to like the people that I work with because I'm probably going to spend more time with them than my own family. A slightly higher salary is no justification for being miserable 40 or more hours a week. Before D-day (May 4, 2010, My Diagnosis Day), I really enjoyed every aspect of whatever job I was doing. I love all of the people I work with and really did get up in the morning (most of the time—we all have bad days) and looked forward to what was going to happen next. I kind of feel like everything was just falling into place for me in so many ways and then this happens. I learned to say no to projects that I knew I wouldn't enjoy. More importantly, I love everyone I work with and, being an independent contractor, I work with a lot of people.

My point here is that I think part of the "why is this happening to me?" phases happen because I miss, or am grieving for, my life before breast cancer. I miss walking into the regional center or one of the hospitals and talking with my co-workers. Although, for the most part, I don't go out on weekends with people at work or other things like that, but there is that connection. The email I received from a co-worker yesterday made me realize how important those connections are. I never would have imagined all of the support I have received from everyone going through this. I know in the past when I know that someone is going through a hard time, I will send them an email, a voicemail, whatever, just to let them know I'm thinking about them. Until now, I never realized how much that really meant. The emails or check-ins I get from people are usually just at the right time. All from people that are in my life for this moment. Many times people come into our lives for just a season and then we never really talk with them again, but in our hearts we are still connected.

Besides having my days of "Cancer Sucks", "I have no hair", etc., I realized that a lot of my "bad moments" come from missing the usual day-to-day banter back and forth with the people I've spent most of my day with. Now, of course, as soon as I'm ready, I plan to be back in action, back at work, and as adorable as ever—just with slightly shorter hair.

Or those "bad days" could be because I'm home more, and being in the house all day drives me nuts. Not to mention that my children are a lot of work. If anyone knows how to get dry erase marker out of fabric blinds, please contact me.

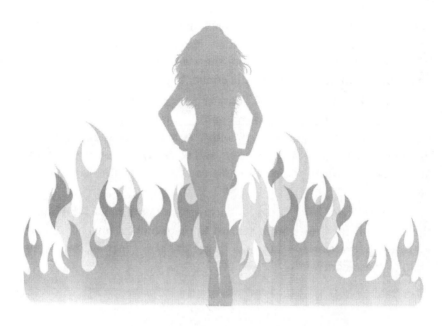

19 SURPRISE SURGERIES &
SMALL SLIPS

August 8-9, 2010

Where to begin? It has been a long week, needless to say. It all started last Tuesday. My right breast incision was starting to turn red and was looking a little bruised. I showed my husband in the morning and he said, "Yeah, it's starting to look red." Since I have had my expanders in my right breast, ironically, the one without the cancer has bothered me. If you recall, I had to have it stitched up because the incision had opened. Anyway, I went about my day and by the evening, it was even more red. My husband told me I needed to go to the emergency room. I was not in the mood for that, mostly because my surgeon is on the other side of the city and not at the closest hospital. I said if it's worse in the morning, that I would call.

I called my doctor's office and, of course, my surgeon was out for the day, so they put me on for his regular day, Thursday. My loving mother and husband said that this was unacceptable, and I needed to call back and get in right now. I called back my surgeon's office and told the

90

receptionist my dilemma. She said to come right in and that one of my surgeon's associates would see me. So, off I went to the doctor's office. When I got there, I told the staff that I just wanted to come and visit because I hadn't been there in two weeks.

The receptionist led me back to my usual room. I could have sworn that I saw my name on the door since I have been there so much. The visits have become as routine as walking into my own bedroom, and I could very well walk into the doctor's office now and take my shirt off while still talking. Vanity and modesty seem to go out the window when every appointment consists of showing your breasts. My surgeon's associate came in the room. Okay. He could definitely qualify for at least a percentage of Dr. McDreamy. He must be like a foot taller than my plastic surgeon. My mood was temporarily lifted since I had something nice to look at. Dr. McDreamy takes one look at my breast and says, "Well, it's infected and we are going to have to take out the mesh holding the expander or the whole expander right away."

Right away meant that afternoon. Great.

The problem with surprise surgeries is the logistics of my life—or anyone's life. Surprise surgeries mean that the condition will decide your timeline. It will decide your priorities. It will choose which meetings to skip and which events to cancel. And right then, a new change meant calling my husband to arrange for childcare for the kids. I had to call and cancel an appointment I had with the state that had been in the books for weeks. I had to call my oncologist's office to let them know what was going on. Everything was back at square one.

The worst thing about surprise surgery when you have cancer is— how is this going to screw up my chemo schedule? Now remember, I was originally thinking chemotherapy would only be for four cycles or eight weeks—now it's six sessions three weeks apart—meaning treatment until October. Surgery may mean I have to postpone chemo, which I'm not excited about. I mean, sure I'm feeling better because the toxins from the last cycle are probably out of my system and I will have another week of feeling good—oh, but wait—if I have surgery—there's recovery time for that. So, I do not yet know how this is going to affect my scheduled chemotherapy on Wednesday, August 11, 2010. So the next couple of days should be interesting.

Next, the surgeon's staff lets me know that they already called over to the emergency room where I will be checking in. I had to move my car so that it wouldn't get lost in the office complex. The emergency room turned out to be about a block away. The waiting room was quite nice, if I might add. The hospital is very old and not in the greatest part of town, but they remodeled the whole thing. Just my luck, I get behind some unbathed crackhead wearing slippers who is having trouble breathing—while holding her pack of cigarettes. Sometimes, you just have to shake your head. Checking in was easy since I was already in their system. I thought the woman was going to hand me a frequent flyer card. Of course, when I get back to triage, the girl knows nothing about me. I let her know that the charge nurse knows and that was why I was sent to the ER instead of the admissions department. She was nice enough to actually figure out what was going on instead of sending me somewhere else. Again, sometimes I'm amazed at how nice people can be.

I was led back to ER and they pretty much brought me back to the pre-operative department. I couldn't believe it—especially having worked in hospitals and surgery centers. The surgeon must have either had time on his hands or they were afraid my breast was going to burst at any moment.

As I'm getting prepped, Dr. Slightly Less Than Dr. McDreamy comes in to tell me about the surgery. I, of course, ask, "Okay, are you in a good mood? It's 3pm. Do you need some coffee? You have done this before, right?" Then the anesthesiologist comes in to go through his speech. I ask him the same things. I tell him no crossword puzzles during surgery. I made sure that he didn't have a fight with his wife or the surgeon in the last 24 hours. Then, I tell him I want to be out for the whole thing. I want to know nothing. I don't want to be on *Jerry Springer* about how I was awake through the whole procedure. I go through all of this with these medical professionals and, of course, they look at me weirdly. Then I tell them that I used to help run a surgery center and know some of the antics that happen during surgery. They tend to look at me differently then, which I'm sure surprises them because without hair and no makeup, I really look like a child.

The surgical nurse comes in to give me my happy cocktail shot that I thought was supposed to put me out. No, it was just the "relaxation shot." So, I got wheeled into the operating room awake. I hate that. I'm still awake while they start strapping me down to the bed, securing my arms, etc. At that point, I asked everyone in the room if they were in a good mood and were all getting along. I then told the sleepy time doctor, the surgery Bartender, that I was ready to be put out. I don't remember anything after that.

The next thing I know is that I'm in recovery. I just love recovery because that is when the doctors come in and tell you what they did and how everything went. Of course, I'm still under heavy sedation, so I didn't hear about half of it. Essentially, the expander was infected on both sides and had to come out. They had me wrapped up in a giant ace bandage. All I could see from that point is that I had one lump on the left side and none on the right side along with my favorite—the drain. I have to say the drains after surgery are the worst because they are giant tubes inserted into the surgical site to allow any excess drainage. It does not feel good and for about a week, I have a tube with a bulb on it that shows attractive gunk. The beauty pageant applications are going to have to be put on hold for a while.

Since my operation was so late in the day, I was staying the night. They wheeled me up to the floor—not med/surgery, but the oncology unit. Yeah, really feeling like a cancer victim at this point. Apparently, while in surgery, they took cultures of whatever infection was in my breast—so those were growing in petri dishes in the lab. Luckily, I had my handy dandy port-o-cath, so IVs went there instead of my hand. I was started on apparently the strongest antibiotic they have and a choice of pain medications. I actually was not in much pain, but who can turn down a Vicodin after surgery? Just seems impolite. My husband left some things for me and then had to attend to the children. I have to say that the nice thing about being in the hospital is the peace and quiet from the chaos at home. My husband had brought my sound machine that I sleep with so I was good to go.

The next morning, I was visited by the hospitalist. I'm not clear of their function except to organize the patients' cases. He saw me for about two minutes. It was at that point I was told that I could be there for a few days because they had to let the cultures grow out to make sure that they send me home with the right antibiotics. Great. Again, who knows how long I'm going to be in the hospital?

Between this time and when my surgeon comes in to see me, I have a look at my scar through the ace bandage. Okay, I have to admit, I started to cry hysterically. It looks awful—at least to someone who is apparently not a plastic surgeon. So, now I have an over-inflated left breast expander on one side and skin and bone on the other—oh yeah, let's not forget I'm bald and have no makeup (my husband forgot the one thing I can't live without—you got it—mascara). When my surgeon comes in, I can't help it and burst into tears asking him if he's sure he's going to be able to do something with it. He takes a look at it and goes on and on about how good it looks. Poor guy. He had to run around the room to look for a tissue for me. In reality, even to a person like me, the stitches look good and not all red or anything. But the way it looks—I can't even describe it. I ask him for a prosthesis in the meantime, since I might be this way until October or later. He actually wrote out a prescription for it, so I assume that insurance will cover part of it. I guess I will be able to take a breast out when someone asks.

I ask my wise surgeon, "What are the chances of the infection going into the other breast?" Guess what his answer was? "I don't know. There is no guarantee." Just what I wanted to hear. Later, I got to thinking, then why didn't they just take both of them out while I was under to risk any further infection and to make me even? The skin is obviously stretched out if they weren't worried about taking out the expander on the left. Of course, in my emotional state, I didn't think to ask, but I will. Who knows? Maybe I will have to have another expander after chemo and they are just not letting me know.

Lola, my nurse for two whole days—that was nice having some consistency in care during one of my emotional breakdowns—was so sweet. She told me that this plastics group is actually one of the best in the city. Her mother was in a car accident and almost lost her ear. They reconstructed it and she said you can hardly tell. That's pretty good. I can't imagine that the ear is an easy thing to reconstruct. With breast reconstruction, you just make sure they are round and perky. Well, and symmetrical and not Frankenstein-like. Okay, fine, I'm sure they are both not easy things to do.

On Friday, my surgeon said that nothing was growing in the cultures and, surgically, I was fine to go home. I ask him, if nothing was growing in the cultures, what could it have been? Guess what his answer was? "I don't know."

However, since I have been on the Superman antibiotic for several days, anything that was there should be gone. I don't know about you, but these vague answers physicians give are really not reassuring—and my surgeon went to Harvard. What was this mysterious cancer and now mysterious infection that chose my body of all bodies? Why was I being chosen by the lottery of illness and not the lottery of millions? One starts to think of the game of chance when they get put into these situations. But I don't know why I'm surprised; I work with a bunch of surgeons and often get the same answer at work. When it has to do with me, I prefer a specific answer. It's humbling to be in the patient's shoes.

My surgeon had not connected with my oncologist at this point, so chemo is still up in the air for this week. I just have to be cleared by the hospitalist. Really? You mean the guy who didn't even touch me and spoke to me for about two minutes and 4 seconds. Apparently, the hospitalist clears people "medically."

Many hours later, the eminent hospitalist shows up. Again, he doesn't touch me. He says that I was breathing, and thus my heart must be beating. Great logic.

He then says, "Your surgeon says you can go home, so I guess we can let you go home on some antibiotics. I'll send you home with some pain medicine and Bactrim."

I think that is the name of it, but whatever—it's a sulfa drug. Again, not wanting to be impolite, I said yes to the pain medicine, but I reminded him that I'm allergic to sulfa drugs—did he even read my chart?

Then he said, "I will have to think about what to send you home with then, and ask your surgeon."

I sarcastically say, "You're the doctor, you mean you don't have some other options in your head?"

Thankfully, he was humorless and didn't get my humor-veiled insult. But the typical care I get, compared to this, seemed like a fairytale.

Then he leaves, and that is it. After what seemed like an eternity, the nurse comes in to give me my discharge papers and my prescriptions. She was very nice and went over them. I got not just one antibiotic, but two, one pain killer, and one prescription for a fake breast. I can't say that I didn't leave with parting gifts. I did leave the pressure thigh-high stockings though. Every time I looked at them I thought of Bubba down in pre-op wearing them. Not a pretty picture.

In the meantime, I have to wait for my husband to come and pick me up because Friday was "Meet your teacher" day at school for the kids. It's hard to believe my cancer adventure starting when the kids were still in school in May. My daughter broke from the crowd, followed the maze of hallways, only to go back to her preschool room. She put her backpack where she used to hang it and sat down like she was ready for school. Apparently, it took much coaching to lure her into her new kindergarten room. My son, on the other hand, was already flirting with the girls in his new room. Which is good because a week ago, he informed us that he heard on the news that there was no school this year because the school fell into a giant hole.

Once I got home, I promptly took a nap since even my sound machine in the hospital didn't mask the techs coming in to take my vitals. Hospital floors can be surprisingly noisy at night. I think someone died on my floor one of the nights, because I heard a long *beeeeeeeeep* and people rushing around. Since I have been home, my kids have been fascinated with the drain. My daughter keeps trying to take it. I had a fanny pack from the last surgery, but I can't find it. I suppose I threw it out thinking I would never need it again.

Finally, while I was in the hospital, I changed my voicemail to say that I was out of the office. My mother said that in my message I sounded like death warmed over. I assume that people are going to leave messages so I can call them up when I'm back in the office, but I had one weight loss surgery patient burn up my phone and leave like three messages each day. I don't think they were planning to have her "emergency" weight loss surgery for several weeks, so the multiple messages was a little overkill.

The past couple of days I have been trying to relax and "recover," if you will. I will be calling both the surgeon and the oncologist tomorrow to see what the status of chemo is this week and to get this dang drain out of my side. I will probably have to get my prosthesis this week also. My white t-shirts are just not the same without two mounds.

■

After my fabulous tour of the hospital last week, I have been waiting in anticipation to see if I'm going to be able to have chemotherapy on Wednesday. It kind of sounds weird WANTING chemotherapy, but if it gets postponed, that means I'm dealing with this *that* much longer. Of course, my surgeon said it should be okay and chemo will probably happen. However, after my initial little "talk" with him about the difference between "uncomfortable" and unbearable pain, I think he is afraid to be anything but positive with me. After all, he is shorter than me—I could probably take him on a good day.

Anyway, I went to the oncologist's office this morning to have my Monday morning blood draw (I know, I have such a lovely schedule). I talked with the PA about the whole situation. He was very positive and said that as long as the incision is clean and not infected, we can probably count on chemo on Wednesday. I told him what meds they gave me when I left the hospital. However, with today's technology, he could just look up the hospital database and see what I was taking and what I left with—remember the parting gifts from yesterday I mentioned? I cleverly hid the drain that is still in my side. This is not scheduled to come out until Thursday. I was kind of thinking that if I have a drain in, which is technically an open area in my skin, that chemo would be out. The PA assured me that he would talk with Dr. Perky and let me know, but for now chemo on Wednesday is on. Wahoo! I also needed to know because I have to pick up the $350 pills I take the days around chemo. I can think a lot of other things I can spend that kind of money on; however, I'm grateful to have insurance.

In the meantime, there is a very small opening on my sutures from my surgery last week. Really nothing, but if you pull it you can see flesh under the skin. I'm sure that is not how it's supposed to look. However, being industrious, I taped it together. Very medical like of myself, if I do say so. I'm rejoicing about being able to proceed with chemo when I call my mother aka Nurse Hatchet, and she tells me to call Dr. Plastic Surgeon right away to see if I need to have the suture looked at, especially if chemo is scheduled for Wednesday. I call Dr. Plastic Surgeon and since it's a Monday morning, I get the answering machine because they are on the phone with 15 people wanting their weekly Botox injections.

I happily, and very tiredly, go home to take a nap. My kids started school today so I would have the house all to myself for at least two hours. I had to get up early to get them out the door. That was rough. While I'm resting my eyes, guess who calls? Dr. Perky oncologist's office. It's the PA. He tells me that he finally got a chance to talk with Dr. Perky herself and she said that since I'm still on the two oral antibiotics from the surgery, I have to wait until I'm through with them. If I don't, the chemo will make any little remaining infection blow up. So no chemotherapy on Wednesday.

Of course, I made various threats to the PA, like falling on the floor and crying and other such things, but unfortunately, Dr. Perky is right. Not to mention that I still have the drain. I mentioned that I hid that from the PA when I was in the office. He sort of laughed and said that I was pretty good because he didn't notice it. Seeing that I was quite upset by this delay, he said he would call Dr. Perky one more time later in the day and see what he could do. I'm thinking, "You're the PA. If Dr. Perky says no chemo for a week, then it's no chemo for a week." Again, the PA trying to save face with me.

Interestingly, later during the day, Dr. Perky's office called me back. The PA chickened out on calling me himself to let me know my chemo had to be rescheduled. He had one of the medical assistants do it. I told the MA who I spoke with to tell the PA that I will try to stop the evil thoughts I was sending his way for getting my hopes up for chemo.

Dr. Plastic Surgeon's office finally called back. I have them now calling me saying, "Hi, how is our favorite patient?" I told them that chemo was off until I was finished with the antibiotics. Unless the small opening gets worse, I have an appointment with Dr. Plastic Surgeon on Thursday to have my drain taken out and to possibly have a few stitches.

In conclusion, I have more doctors' appointments. This cancer thing is really a full-time job. Dang. I don't think I have ever been to the doctor so much. I mean, I have appointments almost every day. I guess I should look on the positive side. I have another full week of feeling halfway decent—except for healing from the surgery. But instead, I did have to take time to mope and cry that I will be bald for longer and this feels like another setback. But don't worry, I didn't let it last all day— otherwise I would not have written today. But still, it sucks. Have I mentioned lately that cancer sucks? Oh, needless to say, I was not in the mood for getting fitted for a prosthesis today. I'm sure that will be a big story by itself.

20 ANOTHER DAY AT THE OFFICE

Having cancer—or any other chronic illness for that matter—is a full-time job. Although I didn't get chemotherapy yesterday, despite my attempts to charm the staff at the Cancer Center, I still had to meet with the PA for my appointment. So, off to work I went. If you think about it, being the popular patient at a cancer center really isn't something to aspire to in the usual realm of things. But since I'm one of the more favorite patients, I get hour-long or longer appointments.

When I get called back, I have to get my vitals checked. Ugh, that means the scale. I guess losing a breast (from the surgery last week) has its advantages. I'm down 10 pounds from where I started before diagnosis. However, this is not a diet plan I would recommend. Also, my blood pressure was low. I'm usually a solid 120/80 girl. The medical assistant leads me back to one of the consultation rooms and goes over my medications and such. She asked if I was having any depression or anxiety. I had to laugh. Well, yeah. I had a string of comments to make about that, but I kept them to myself. My mother would be so proud about that. She also asked if I was more fatigued than usual or dizzy, and you know what? I have been. The fatigue has been killing me, but the past couple of days I have actually been dizzy and out of breath. And I can't account that to meeting the men of *Grey's Anatomy*.

After being grilled about the same things that I usually get grilled about, the PA finally arrives. I think Dr. Perky was at a conference. But I have to say for all of you biased nurse practitioners out there (I'm one of them myself), he is actually really knowledgeable. Anyway, he explains again why I couldn't have chemo that day. Then he goes over my bloodwork with me. This is a long conversation because I really don't know what it all means. The good news is that my white blood cell count is in normal range. The bad news is that my hemoglobin and red blood cells are low—so low that I have mild chemotherapy-induced anemia. This accounts for the dizziness and constant fatigue. (This is from my mother's explanation). Apparently hemoglobin carries oxygen to the brain—mine is low so I'm not getting enough oxygen to the old noggin. This may also account for my low blood pressure. Now get this: my hemoglobin is at a 10—whatever that means—apparently on the low side, but not low enough for insurance to pay for a shot that would significantly help this problem. If I had a 9.9, the insurance will pay for the shot.

The PA anticipates that this number will continue to drop. I looked it up online but 60-70 percent of chemo patients get this. And the fabulous PA said that if it gets too bad, I would have to have a blood infusion! I said, "You mean get SOMEONE else's blood?!"

He assured me they type and cross-match it beforehand. But still, what if I get someone's blood who is not as adorable as myself? That would not be good. Can you imagine? Basically, as long as nothing else goes wrong between now and next Wednesday, I should be back on track for chemo, which of course feels like it's going to last the rest of my life.

One last discussion we had is about the strength of the chemotherapy I'm on. I told him that some ladies next to me at my last hydration were calling Adriamycin the "Red Devil" and how you don't want it. I mentioned that to him, and he basically said it's an older but effective medication, but with that medication and the other two, I'm on probably one of the more toxic regimes. My toxicity level was beyond my very own humanity, I thought. The body is truly strong to survive the onslaught of first cancer, and now this "Red Devil", which can apparently eat away at the skin. That's why the nurse is so careful when she injects it. If I was her, I'd put on a bodysuit. Just another happy thought. It makes you wonder, if it eats your skin, what is it doing when it goes into your veins? I'll let the medical people ponder that one.

After that appointment, I had to come home and meet with the woman who is going to be the kids' case manager for Department of Developmental Disabilities—finally, after six months of trying to get services. My son was denied. My daughter was approved. By the time that appointment was over, I was ready for my daily nap. One of the perks of this job.

■

Today "at work", I had my plastic surgeon appointment. Again, being the favorite patient, I got there early and the receptionist brought me in first before another couple that walked in at their exact appointment time. Dr. Plastic Surgeon came in and took out my drain from the surgery. I hate that thing. He said that my incisions looked good. I did ask, "Now, as long as you were in there, why not just take out the other expander?" He gave me a number of reasons. But the real news is that, although the incision was on my right breast, where the expander was removed has lots of skin for the reconstruction—it's possibly not enough. I might have to have ANOTHER expander placed before reconstruction.

I knew it. I heard him say that really fast and quietly in the hospital but wasn't sure I heard him correctly because of all of the drugs I was on! But again, he assured me that since most of the area is stretched out, I would not need the expander for long..

Dr. Plastic Surgeon asked if I had gone to get my prosthesis yet. I told him I didn't want to go until after this appointment because I wanted to make sure my sutures were okay. Also, I have a feeling that is probably going to be an emotional day. All the women who run it are cancer survivors. The last cancer survivor who gave me a hug when we did the "second opinion" Cancer Center consultation made be completely emotional. Yeah, again, those questions the medical assistant asks like, "Are you feeling depressed or anxious?" Come on. Anyone with any emotions who is going through all of this is going to be depressed and anxious. I can say that, not just as a patient but as a psychologist! And anxious—now that I know that the "Red Devil" eats your skin—yeah, a bit nervous that the nurse on Wednesday is not going to be in a good mood so she doesn't get any on me or her. We want our chemo nurses very happy.

So my "job" will continue tomorrow. However, like any job, when you get home, there is the rest of the family to attend to. I have to find people for services for my daughter. Dentists for both of the kids. You know, the usual daily stuff. Interestingly, that doesn't go away just because you have cancer.

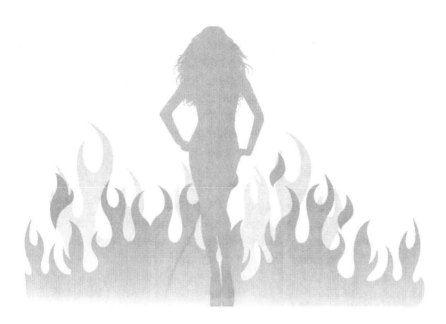

21 THIRD CHEMO TREATMENT

August 16-19, 2010

So far, it looks like I will have my third chemo treatment on Wednesday—unless I get a call that my white blood cell count is too low, which I think is impossible given that I have been on the heavy duty and most expensive antibiotics since surgery. Of course, I still have the low iron, but the hope is that went down because then the insurance will pay for the "big shot". Kind of reminds me of the weight loss surgery patients—if they just gain 10 more pounds, they will be eligible for surgery.

This weekend was all about stocking up in anticipation of not feeling good after chemo. Of course, that meant a Costco trip. You should never go there when you're hungry. Big mistake. I don't know how the stuff adds up so quickly. I actually tried to follow through with my treatment plan of leisure skills this weekend. Costco counts, in my opinion, but I started to read a book. Wow. I know. The excitement. The thrill. I had to resist doing work. I did okay until Sunday afternoon, when I couldn't take it anymore and did some work. I have a long way to go.

Today was the usual Monday morning blood draw, then I went to the place where they have the prosthesis. I actually walked in to make an appointment for a fitting. I wanted to scope out the place to see if I was going to be a freak about it or not. Guess who runs the front? Pink ladies, aka old lady volunteers, but they wear blue jackets now. Everything in the store seemed geared for the more "mature" women. They had cotton dress-like pajamas that I think I have only seen on *Leave it to Beaver* or *Little House on the Prairie*. Right next to that, they have "lubrication" products. Yes, what you're thinking I'm talking about is what it's for. Even if I was going to buy something like that, I don't think I would have the nerve to bring them up to the 101-year-old lady at the counter. A non-volunteer woman came out to take me in the back to make the appointment for this week. They actually have "fitters", and the appointments take about an hour. Behind her was a wall with prostheses in boxes lined up to the wall. All kinds. Some of them even had "sagging" lines on them. Ugh. That should be a fun visit. I was wearing my baseball hat, so the woman asked if I was there for a wig also. I said, "No." I almost felt out-of-style there. I have the wig, I just haven't had the nerve to wear it yet.

I also had to go around to the various pharmacies and pick up my hundreds of dollars' worth of prescriptions before Wednesday. The loose change I get from stripping with only one breast doesn't pay for all of it, so I'm glad that insurance picks up at least some of the tab.

Speaking of cost. I just got the "bill" from my emergency hospital stay. The hospital is charging my insurance $27,000.00. That's just for the hospital, not the surgeon or the anesthesiologist. Again, I have pretty much met my deductible, but still. I'm so thankful I have insurance, otherwise they might be using Scotch tape or a fishing line instead of sutures and Ziploc baggies for the expanders. Also, one of my chemo visits was about $12,000.00 for all of the medications. After all of this money spent on my body, I would hope that I would at least turn out like Jennifer Aniston. But instead, I'm bald, pale from low iron, and have various scar marks from surgeries, blood tests, and the culprit: cancer. On the bright side, I'm probably more interesting to look at. I must be, because I often get stared at more than before.

■

Yesterday was my third of six chemo treatments. I'm over the hump, I suppose. I don't feel as great as I did after the last two treatments. It didn't take as long to get the medicines. I think they speed things up once they think that you can handle it because usually I'm the last patient to leave the facility! I'm also happy to report that my adoring husband sat with me the entire time and brought me movies and lunch. It was a rather dreary group there. One woman sitting next to me was on her third cycle of three chemo treatments. In other words, this was the third time she was going through all the cycles. I didn't really ask anymore, but sometimes people who have cancer just want to tell you their whole story. I had to come home and take a nap this time, and usually I'm feeling really great for at least three days after the treatment because of all of the happy pills they give you, but not this time. I cancelled my prosthesis appointment for today because I thought that I wouldn't be able to go after having two appointments this morning.

This morning, I got the "happy shot" that is supposed to up my white blood cell count since chemo tears them down. The bummer is that my daughter came home with a cold last week. My nadir period—the time when my white blood cells are the lowest—should be about next Wednesday before the shot kicks in. I'm really hoping that the kids don't bring home any more viruses at that point. By next week, pending everything goes well, I should have my entire schedule of chemo outlined for me until the end.

My next stop of the morning was to my actual breast cancer surgeon. I haven't seen her since I had my port installed. She was the one who got everything moving so quickly. It's so interesting how each doctor has different bedside mannerisms. Dr. Plastic Surgeon is really sweet, but not good at giving bad news. Dr. Perky says everything is going to be fine. Dr. Breast Cancer Surgeon is very caring, but conservative. She said that she was very concerned when she found out that my right expander was infected because it's so close to the port. Remember the port? The one that I just found out goes right to my heart. Yeah, we really don't want that getting infected. I mentioned to Dr. Breast Cancer Surgeon that Dr. Perky wants my ovaries out and will refer me to an OB/GYN. Dr. Breast Cancer Surgeon suggested that I consider having the whole works out—a total hysterectomy—as long as they were taking out the ovaries. (Oh boy. Can you feel my pulse racing?) And that it should be done before I have the breast reconstruction because the breast reconstruction will be a lot more recovery time. Also, I may need to have a new expander put in where they took it out. Great. That means at least three to four more surgeries, if everything goes right, by the end of the year.

I also asked her about the shadow they saw on the PET scan. Of course, she said "I don't know; we'll cross that bridge when we get to it."

I guess I will have all of those tests again after chemo to determine if there is anything there. So far no one seems to be worried about it. But you hate to have that hanging over your head. Dr. Breast Cancer Surgeon also wants to consult with Dr. Plastic Surgeon to make sure that the surgery will go well. I love how she's on top of everyone. Since the fabulous scar that was left from taking the expander was skin-sparing, it looks awful. She even kind of admitted it. But I guess a new expander will help that. I had to laugh because she asked if I wanted to be big and maybe that is why he overfilled me. I said NO. I'm not looking for double D's, despite my husband's pleas.

Needless to say, it's been a hectic two days. Cancer still sucks. I just have to remember that this is one season in my life and maybe the lesson is to slow down. But, knowing myself, I'm sure that I will be off and running once this is all over.

It was funny, when I was in the lobby today one of the other patients was talking to me about her experience. Apparently she had to have chemo first before reconstruction because her tumor was so big. She was still trying to work as much as she could. That would really suck if I knew that the tumor was still in me. But one thing she said, which I have said before, is that the problem with the cancer treatment is that it takes away your life for a while. You really miss it as you sit in the prison of chemo appointments, consultations, and follow-ups. Even the days I dreaded going into the office, knowing I was going to hear the same stories or do the same assessments, I felt alive. I know I will get there again. But the current fatigue, nausea and full-time job of doctors' visits is going to make that an impossibility for a while. For now, being a patient has become my new career.

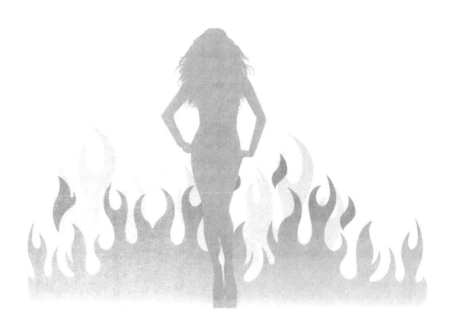

22 LOW WHITE CELL BLOOD COUNT

August 26-31, 2010

I *was* feeling pretty good today until the Cancer Center called me to tell me that my white blood cell level was so low that I need to take "precautions" through the weekend. If I get a slight fever or the chills, I need to go to the ER right away. Also, my hemoglobin was actually low enough that I was able to go in for the expensive shot that insurance only pays for if your levels are really low. The Cancer Center hasn't called me before to tell me how low my WBC was, so I started to kind of freak out about it. I've been using hand sanitizer like crazy and taking my temperature constantly. I kind of anticipated this, so I didn't go to the kids Back to School Night last night, which I felt bad about, but now it turns out it was a good thing. I got a fax of my bloodwork, and it said "critical" under the levels for WBC and another level. I have never seen "critical" on a lab work-up before, so I guess it's isolation for me in the house all weekend. It's weird when you let your mind start thinking about all of the germs out there. One of the new nurses at the Cancer

Center shook my hand and I had to go wash it right away.

I have been a bit of a freak show about that I'm now Miss Anti-Germ. I love the smell of bleach in the morning. Ironically, I might just become like my uncle and brother who have holsters on their belts for various cleaning products.

On the other hand, when I was at the Cancer Center, one of the newer medical assistants told me I looked beautiful and natural. Of course, keep in mind that I have no hair and wear a baseball cap everywhere. She was very nice about it. Apparently, I was the discussion of the moment because the other MA joined in. She told me that if they ever wanted a "cancer poster child", I would be it because I look so healthy and my skin looks good. She laughed and said that she wasn't sure if she should tell me that because she didn't want me to think that I was hitting on her.

Obviously, she meant it as a compliment. But what exactly do you say when someone says you should be the cancer poster child? I was quite speechless. I did thank her because I have been asking everyone if I have that sallow skin color going on and now I know that I don't. Yeah, I think that one is going to go into "Really?" category.

Then again, how does one compliment a cancer patient? "Gee, you don't look so pale today." Because seriously, I look like a cancer patient. I know. I get the looks at Target, the drive-thru, etc. The compliment from my mom was that my voicemail message doesn't sound like I'm at death's door anymore. I guess I won't be changing that anytime soon. My husband also tells me wonderful things, but I didn't expect the cancer poster child thing. Ah, the new and exciting experiences I'm having. It's hard to be incognito at this point.

■

After getting the news about my critically low white blood cell count, I have been basically in isolation and house-bound for the last week. I would like to report that in that time, I will have written the great American novel—it should be on bookshelves next month—developed my own television show—starring me, but with hair—and solved world hunger. I also cleaned, organized the entire house, and sewed the kids a completely new wardrobe of my own designs. I *would* like to report this, but, alas, I cannot. My imagination can get the best of me.

Ever notice when you have downtime, you always have the best intentions of getting things done, but for some reason it does not happen? Well, this time, my excuse takes the cake. These damn chemo treatments actually cause side effects like fatigue, dizziness, and brain fog—and remember, I'm blonde to begin with—you can tell from my eyebrows, which are still intact.

Most of my week was actually spent getting done what work I could do and then taking my daily nap. I'm beginning to love the afternoon nap. I can see why many countries take a "siesta" in the afternoon. It's oh-so-refreshing and allows me to be more together and less fatigued for when the kids get home. Being that is the week before my next treatment, I actually feel pretty good and have not required the extra sleep. However, the problem with feeling good is that I tend to overdo it. On Sunday, I was feeling slightly fatigued and occasionally winded throughout the day, but had moments of delusion that I was 100%. I started to move at my usual pace as I was bringing one of the kids a bowl of popcorn and tripped up the stairs. I fell on my knee and bent my little finger back. For a minute, I thought for sure I had broken both my knee and my finger. My darling husband cleaned up the popcorn and demanded that I go take a seat and slow down.

Luckily, my knee is fine and I think I just sprained my finger. This is the same hallway, of course, in which I broke my elbow this past February. Yeah, maybe walking needs to be on my treatment plan. This incident wiped me out and I was back on the couch. So much for being Super Girl. The rest of Sunday was spent watching old movies with my husband, much to his delight. I don't usually like to watch old movies, but he does. I actually really enjoyed some of them. Of course, when a black and white one was on, I had to ask, "Why isn't it in color?" just to annoy my husband. Since film is his thing, questions like this aggravate him to no end.

On Monday, I did finally leave the house to take the dog to the vet. Quite the adventure, seeing as I haven't left the house in about a week. However, I'm amazed at how such an outing can be so tiring. I went looking like my cancer victim self and the staff seemed overly friendly. It's hard to tell these days if someone is being extra nice.

Anyway, going to the vet is kind of like going to the dentist. You know when the dentist questions you about flossing and you're in a dilemma about if you're going to lie about it or not because he is going to figure it out once he examines your teeth anyway? The vet that we go to looks like a spa for dogs. My last apartment wasn't as nice as this place. Molly, our Chihuahua, was trembling the whole time. We get the brand new vet—I know because there was a picture of her in the exam room outlining her credentials and newness. One of her special interests is the "Human-animal bond." Great—I get the vet who is the equivalent to a tree hugger for animals.

She is concerned about how much Molly is shaking and wants to know if I "get her out and socialize her with other dogs." She goes on to say how much I should probably get her out more and this kind of nervousness she's displaying in the exam room probably would go away. She gives me the lecture on "clicker trainer". Again, my mother would be proud of me that I didn't say what I was really thinking as she was giving me the low down on "socializing" my seven-pound dog. Really? Do I look like socializing my dog is high on my priority list? She even suggested that I could bring Molly by the vet (without an appointment) to socialize. It was all I could do not burst out laughing.

I'm sorry. I love our dog and I'm a dog lover, but carving out time in my day and actually penciling in "doggie play date" in my calendar seems absurd at this point. "Okay, let's look at the week. Doctor's appointment, blood draw, kids' homework, setting up therapy for the kids, doggie play date, chemo." Yeah, not happening. The actual vet appointment where procedures were performed probably could have taken a total of 10 minutes instead of 45. Guess they want to make sure I get my money's worth. After the appointment, again, I was surprisingly drained. So was Molly, by the way. She slept the rest of the day.

∎

The chemo nurse who's been treating me since the beginning told me last week, when I went in for my injection of superpowers, that she'd given her two-week notice the week before. Apparently, since I'm one of the "favorite patients" she told me that there has been a lot of turnover at the Cancer Center. Frankly, I wasn't surprised because she is the only chemo nurse and works her butt off because she's the only one in the room who can access the port and actually give the IV medications. She told me that due to the "higher ups", things are a bit unorganized. She probably shouldn't have told me this, but having helped run surgery centers, I know what she means. There is always drama in medical practices. I had no idea until I started to do more medical psychology. That's why there are so many medical dramas on television, because there is that much drama—and I'm not talking about the patients—usually it's the staff.

Anyway, I know this, but as a patient I didn't really need to hear that.

Great. So, for my next chemo treatment, I'll be questioning the new nurse, "Um, are you sure that's the right stuff that you're pumping into my port that goes directly into my heart?" The thought of not getting chemo administered correctly is a little disconcerting, particularly since I don't just get one chemo medication, I get three. When they put the medication on the IV stand, the bags have a sticker with my name on it. I really don't want to look up and see "Bob Smith" on my IV bag. That would be bad. Luckily, Nurse Hatchet, aka my mother, will be along next week for my chemo. I'm sure she'll be paying attention. I have an appointment with my oncologist on Wednesday and I'll be asking about the staff issues.

Think about it; as patients, we really try to go with the illusion that our doctors know best, but they're human. It's like any other office. When the patient is not within earshot (or sometimes when they are), staff talk, they get distracted, the doctors might have their own issues. I know this because I work with doctors and surgeons. Again, hard to make the switch from provider to patient in these situations. Kind of like when the doctor in the hospital was going to discharge me with a medication I'm allergic to—you need to be on top of these people because, as much as you think your doctor knows you, you're ultimately "the breast cancer patient in Room 412". That's why I use my psychological mind tricks by saying, "It's your favorite patient calling." Of course, a lot of this is because I'm adorable and I probably am their favorite patient, but it's also so that they remember me and I'm not just a chart in the stack.

My next chemotherapy appointment is on September 8th, the day after I turn 40. I can hardly stand to see that in writing! I'm pretty sure that at one point in my life ,I thought most people at age 40 were older than dirt, and now here I am. Of course, at this point, I would rather be 40 than the alternative. I have stopped saying things like, "I'm never going to get old." Seems to have more significance these days. Old doesn't sound too bad.

I think I mentioned that I read about a female psychologist who was in her 90's living in Los Angeles still seeing a few patients a week. Now I'm hoping for that. Or maybe more like Betty White's comeback at 88 years old. I saw a clip where she quipped to a 20-something girl by saying, "You might be a quarter of my age, but I can still take you down." At that age, I will no longer need my filter. Like the poem says, "When I'm an old lady, I shall wear purple." I'm pretty sure at that age I would tell the vet, "Really? Socialize my dog? Did you notice I have no hair and am missing a breast? Did you notice that I look like the albino guy without hair from the movie *Powder*? My dog's social life is not really a big concern right now, but thanks for the tip."

But I guess, to be fair, it goes back to: How does one approach someone who is obviously going through cancer treatment? It's a pretty visible illness at this point. My husband has started having poker parties on Friday nights with some people he met. I haven't had the nerve to go to the "man cave" while these are happening. He explained why his wife is hiding out with the children. One of his guests owns a local hair salon. As they were talking, he was very nice and said to send me over to his salon and he would do my hair. My husband reminded him that I have no hair. Poor guy. He was quite embarrassed. Kind of funny, actually. You have to have a sense of humor with this.

23 CHEMO & CAKE

September 7-9, 2010

This week, I had my "mid-point" meeting with Dr. Perky, the oncologist. I had to have my vitals taken and blood drawn, then I was placed in a room. The MA went over my symptoms again like she always does. Again, she asked about depression and anxiety. I burst out laughing. She smile and says, "Situational?" At least she's beginning to get a sense of humor. She then left the room, telling me to undress from my waist up. The Cancer Center provides nice, silky robes to hang out in while you're in this phase, somehow trying to mask why you're really there.

At this point, I'm thinking about how some of my own patients must feel when they come to see me. Eagerly awaiting albeit patiently for me to come out and call them back. She was about 20 minutes late, but somehow when talking about chemo and cancer, I can stand the wait. In these appointments, I can't help feeling like a little girl waiting for directions or for some type of good news. The PA was also in the room, taking notes and using my case as a teaching situation. She went over my symptoms. I talked about how horrible the hot flashes were and she told me to "go to the old lady aisle of the drug store and get some herbs." No, she didn't really say that, but I can say that I now know what evening primrose oil is. In addition, I've had some back abdominal pain, so I got a prescription for that. My bin of pills is almost overflowing at this point.

At one point in the conversation, Dr. Perky asked if I had any other questions. What do you say? Am I cancer-free yet? Am I cured yet? Can we quit this yet? Do I really need three more rounds of chemo? Ugh! I again ask her, "Now you're sure there is no way to tell if this is working or not? What happens when we're done? There must be some type of test you can take to figure this all out." Again, no, there is no sure way of knowing. I will follow up with her every three months for the first year, and then every six months, and so on. Being a psychologist and having my profession be such an ambiguous science, I kind of expect medicine to be more objective—it's not. I sat there like I was 12 years old, waiting for her to tell me I'm going to be okay. I had to ask her, "Now you're sure they got it all at surgery?" Dr. Perky reassures me that I'm going to be fine, but I'm like Scully on the *X-Files*—I want proof that she just can't seem to provide.

Before my diagnosis, I had made an appointment to see a dermatologist to have my skin looked at. Since I'm so fair, that was part of my old lady plan—to have the "imperfections" on my skin looked at. I had cancelled the appointment when I'd found out I had breast cancer.

I asked Dr. Perky if I should still schedule an appointment—you know—check out for any melanomas, that sort of thing. I thought for sure she would say, "No, not necessary. We have you on such killer stuff that it doesn't make a difference." She didn't. She suggested that I go, if for no other reason so that I don't have more doctor's appointments after this is all over with. Now won't that just suck if I make the appointment and I have skin cancer? I'm going to be positive and not think about it. I'll keep you posted on that one.

The appointment ended with a physical exam. "Ooooh, it's healing so good."

I was like, "Yeah, maybe to an oncologist and plastic surgeon, but to me it looks like Frankenstein boobies."

She assured me that would all be taken care of and that 2011 would be a great year. Now I see how annoying I can be when I'm perky.

Now comes the waiting. I've been feeling really good this past week and am not having to lie in bed all day. I think the shot they gave me for anemia really helped. I feel so good that I'm dreading next week when I have a doctor's appointment every day, including chemo on Wednesday. Every day! Dang.

■

It was a busy week. I had my friend in from Chicago and she spent the weekend, which gave me a bit of normalcy. She actually took my picture, and I threatened to kill her if it ends up on her Facebook. My first picture without hair—but of course, I did have a hat on and a "Princess sash." And then my other friend got a cake that looked like it came right out of *Cake Boss*. It had a shoe on it with a label saying "Adorable One" and a line saying, "Happy Birthday to the Adorable One."

Then Mary Poppins (that's what we call the kids' babysitter because she's so wonderful) got me two full boxes of chocolates from Rocky Mountain Chocolate Factory, and my brother and his wife sent me a bouquet of cookies. Needless to say, I was on a sugar high until I had my chemo yesterday.

I was feeling really good all week before chemo, which I was dreading. Why do I always think that I'm going to get stuff done while I'm sitting there getting these toxic medications that come out in biohazard bags? First they dope you up on "pre-chemo" meds for a while, which make you sleepy. And, like I mentioned, we have a new nursing staff, so I was on extra guard to make sure I was getting everything that I needed. Of course, this time my Mama Bear was along to make sure I got all my needs met. At one point, I had nausea, so we asked for some extra anti-nausea medication. The new nurse took so long getting the medication, I thought that my mom was going to go Shirley MacLaine on her if she didn't get me the medication sooner.

This time, chemo didn't go as well as expected. I got home and my gut was killing me. Stomach cramps and everything. Real bummer. I know that it's all supposed to be cumulative, but still. After feeling so good for a week before chemo, I'm not looking forward to the fatigue, and not the extra bonus of a swollen colon, but apparently it's all part of the course. I'm glad I got all the sugar in before yesterday because I'm already back on the bland diet.

Only two more chemo treatments to go, then we start with the surgeries. The doctors want my ovaries out because having breast cancer gives me more likely a chance of having ovarian cancer sometime in the future. Great. However, my oncologist continues to be encouraged that I'm doing great and that we got to the cancer early enough. Early enough so that I don't need radiation, which is a blessing. Again, I continue to try to figure out what meaning, if anything, this all has to do with my future. I'm sure part of it's needing to slow down and not be so driven by work.

Also, through this I've had so many good friends come out of the woodwork with encouraging emails and voicemails. I can't tell you how much I appreciate that—even if emotionally, I'm not ready to talk in person or on the phone. I appreciate everyone pitching in to help me out.

I'm off to take a nap and hopefully get my "gut" (my mother gave me a lesson on anatomy this morning and it's not my stomach, but my intestinal tract that's bothering me) back on track because that feeling plus lack of sleep will put anyone over the edge.

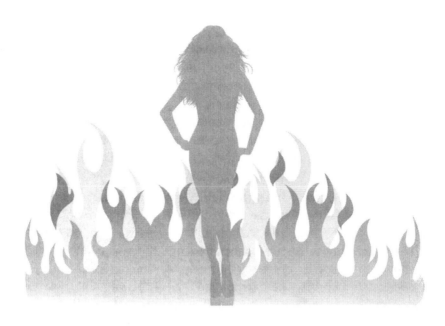

24 FOUR DOWN, TWO TO GO

September 13, 2010

I had my fourth round of chemotherapy. Just two more rounds to go before I finally knock this villain out. The oncologist said it would probably get a little worse, and that I would feel tired. She was right. I have been in bed most of the weekend with gut pain and most of the symptoms from the Taxotere that I didn't get in the first two rounds. This includes flushing, gut pain, and all other sorts of fabulous details I won't bore you with. I really felt icky that first night.

On Friday, I went in for extra fluids to ensure that I was well hydrated for the weekend. Who knew that drinking alone doesn't give you what you need? I have to sit there for about two hours while I get fluids. My mom came with me.

That day, the guy sitting in the chair next to me was telling his story to the woman beside him. He has colon cancer that went to the liver. He's had 24 rounds of chemotherapy. He's also had radiation so drastic that for three days afterward, they kept him isolated and used a Geiger meter to see how close they could get to him. After all of that, the tumors still haven't shrunk. He was there getting some type of medicine that was supposed to help so that the tumors stay where they are.

That kind of story definitely put things in perspective for me. He was about my age and was on the phone talking about taking his kids to sports practice. I guess seeing that one in eight women will experience breast cancer, I'm pretty lucky that it was caught so early. Of course, listening to this guy next to me, I couldn't help but get a little crazy thinking that maybe I need to have every scan on the face of the planet. But I could only face one fear at a time.

I sure am glad that I got all of the chocolate and sweets I did for my birthday and was able to enjoy them before chemo, because I can hardly stand anything stronger than 7-Up at this point. I'm hoping that at least this will be a good weight-loss plan. I mean, my BMI is still within normal limits, but five pounds here and there wouldn't hurt. I do have to put makeup on or else I really look like one of the kids from the St. Jude's commercials. The chemo made my face swell a bit this time. My husband says it's all in my head, but I was paranoid before that I had a big head!

So, if you go out to eat today, please have a nice juicy steak or something spicy for me!

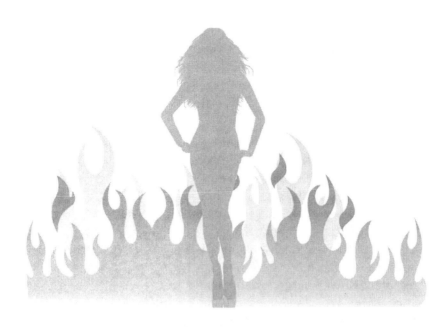

25 FEELING BETTER

September 14, 2010

Good news. I didn't throw up once all day! As a matter of fact, my stomach feels better! This is most excellent, because I still have chocolate left over from my birthday. I sneaked one today—don't tell Nurse Hatchet. I'm still on the wonderful bland diet, but I'm not keeling over in pain. This is such a bonus when you're trying to get things done. This kind of pain reminds me of when I was in college and taking the prep classes for the graduate record exam. One of the reasons I became a psychologist is because I had every psychosomatic problem as a kid— meaning lots of stress-related disorders like Irritable Bowel Syndrome

Tomorrow, I meet with the oncologist again and get my blood count. Any bets as to what my WBC will be and if I will be sequestered to the house again? Of course, my son has had a fever all weekend. Luckily (for me, not for her), Nurse Hatchet has been in to help take care of him so that I don't get the fever.

Another good thing about not having gut pain is that I get to deal with my children. My daughter was up at 4:30am and never went back to bed. She likes to rub her hands across my bald head and then will giggle a little bit. I have to say, I'm getting used to the bald thing. It's very cool when it's hot and, again, showering is a breeze. I spoke to someone else who went through the same type of chemo I'm going through. She finished and she said that about four weeks after the last chemo, she can actually taste things again. Most stuff tastes like cardboard right now—except chocolate. That still tastes good, even when I have to imagine it.

More good news. The kids' bus driver has stopped looking at me like I'm a victim. Everyone has been so nice and supportive. I really think that this is a lesson in patience for me. I'm hyper and am usually doing 100 things at once. This experience has really taught me to slow down and learn that most things are not urgent and one can really prioritize. I still don't think that I will be socializing my dog anytime soon, but I have learned that the world doesn't end because I'm not actively doing something. Remind me of this when this is all over. I figure that this whole process, with surgeries and everything, will probably take until the end of the year. My hyper little brain is already planning how I'm going to fly out of the chute starting in January.

Another bet to take: How will my hair grow out? For some people it grows out curly and gray. Yeah. I don't think I'm going to be into the whole gray thing, but curly might not be bad. After all, I was the Perm Queen of the 1980s. As a matter of fact, when I first moved to Los Angeles, someone asked me if I was from the Midwest because of my "big hair". The last time I had short hair was as a freshman in high school. My brother emailed me a picture of that haircut just the other day.

I've stopped looking up my cancer on the internet. That was getting to be overwhelming. But I will tell you this: The Cancer Center has a certain smell to it. Every time I walk through the door, the smell reminds me of chemo. Not really excited about that—especially since, according to the oncologist, she and I will be buddies for life since I will need regular check-ups. I guess there will always be reminders of this time in my life.

∎

I spoke too soon yesterday; I was not up to par today with my gut pain. But again, when I walked into the doctor's office, there was an emaciated woman in a wheel chair, so I guess I'm doing pretty well.

Before I went to the doctor's office, I had to stop off at Target. To add to the excitement of my day, we went to a different Target than the one by my house. I know. The thrill. I can see that you're jealous. I like to change it up because I think I know all of the cashiers at the local Target.

I'm sure that I'm the "cancer woman". At the new and exciting Target down the road, I get the new girl at the check-out who can't seem to figure out the "magic" of the conveyor belt. I'm standing there, and she is telling me how fickle it is. Well, there was a loaf of bread right in front of the sensor that was causing the belt not to move. Really? Again, another moment where I really want to say something, but I'm working on patience. She takes the loaf of bread and the "magic" begins. Do you ever wonder how many moments of your life are wasted on stuff like that? Not like I was in a hurry, but still. Deep breaths. Deep breaths.

I had my update with the oncologist's PA today. Basically, the good news is that I'm doing well and only have two more chemo treatments to go. Bad news is that most likely I will have more gut and body pain the next two times. Since I had bad gut pain today, I was not happy about that at all. Again, he reminded me that I'm getting a pretty harsh dose of chemo with my three medications. I would really like to have been a fly on the wall when that decision was made. Luckily, my mother was there to ask some of the medication questions that I have no idea about. Good news: The next chemo treatment, I should be getting some more happy drugs like Ativan to help with the pain and nausea. I like happy drugs.

The anticipation of these visits is always more exciting than the actual visit. I'm always hoping that the doctor or PA is going to have some revelation that all of this was some big mistake. But unfortunately, they don't. It's basically, "Yeah, you're going to not feel good. It's chemo. What did you expect?" Then the PA, as we're leaving, says, "Boy, it must feel like this has gone quick. Only two more." I could have slapped him. I said, "No, actually I feel like I've lived a lifetime since May 4."

Sometimes I feel like I'm literally listening to the clock tick. At least the PA could tell me it's going to end. For some patients, I'm sure the consults are more difficult when the cancer is worse.

Driving home from the doctor's office always puts my mind into overdrive. Can my gut pain really just be the chemo? Or did they miss something? Maybe I have polyps on my colon. Maybe something spread and they don't want to tell me. I have to do therapy on myself. Which, by the way, is usually taking a nap. That seems to help, particularly since chemo brain makes it difficult for me to concentrate on anything worthwhile. Remember, I have little to no leisure skills, so if I can't work to keep myself busy because I don't feel well, the choices are limited. Did you know that they have sitcom re-runs on TBS all day long? Yeah, I really got to work on some other leisure activities. I saw one woman knitting during her chemo treatment. But do I really want to learn to knit, scrapbook, needlepoint, etc.? I just am not seeing it. Besides, I'm pretty sure when this is all over, I do not want a thing I knitted from chemo treatments laying around the house. That would be quite the conversation starter, though. "Hey, I knitted this wall hanging in chemo treatment." How would you respond to that?

■

I got my bloodwork back and am sequestered to the house again. My white blood count is 0.8. The nurse called and said the level was "critical" again. At least nothing is boring, and critical meant a new development. She said if I get any type of fever or open wound to go to the emergency room right away. I could get sepsis—a blood disorder that causes you to go into shock! I told her that no one mentioned that to me before. Why do they leave out all of these little details? Or maybe it's the rush of treatment that makes it impossible to list every single possible side effect. All day, I've been bathing in antibacterial lotion. If I had to leave, I guess I could be like this woman I saw at the store yesterday—she was wearing latex gloves while shopping. That was a first. But what an idea.

This again forces me to work on my leisure skills—from home. I have some work I can do, but that's not going to fill up the whole day. I'm trying to make napping a skill, but since the last chemo, that hasn't worked out for me. I can't sleep, either because of hot flashes or gut pain or because my children don't seem to understand that when it's dark out, it's time to sleep. I could take up reading fiction (*gasp!*) but I have never done that. I mean, I have read fiction, but I can probably tell you the two books that I have read. Usually, I'm reading psychology-related books. I know. I'm a psychology geek. I can't help it. Old habit from graduate school.

We did so much reading that the only thing non-school related I would read would be *People* on the train ride home. My idea of fun is reading new articles on Medline, then there's television and movies. My husband has probably more movies than what Blockbuster once had. I don't want to watch something sad, or where people are sick, or war movies. Stuff like that is too depressing. I know, I can be pathetic. I haven't learned the art of vegging out yet.

Obviously, I have issues. And now, I'm stuck in the house to deal with them. Oh well, better than contemplating all of this from a hospital bed!

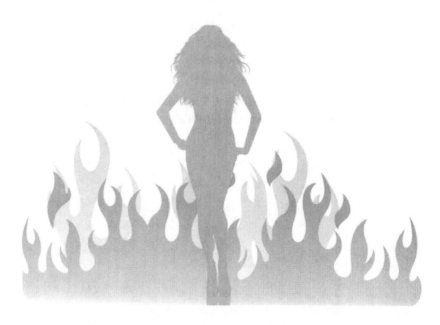

26 FEELING ISOLATED...

AND BALD

September 17-23, 2010

I'm getting used to the bald thing. It really is a time-saver. No shampoo. No conditioner. No mousse. No hairspray. No curling iron. None of that. And I'm cool in the heat. How come this trend has only become popular with balding men who shave all of their hair so they can hide the fact that they're balding? I mean, isn't a man's head of hair just as much a part of their appeal as a woman's?

Imagine Tom Selleck or Johnny Depp completely bald. Oh well, I will savor my baldness for now. I asked the doctor how long after my last chemo will it take for it to start growing back—and she said TWO MONTHS!I was thinking like three weeks. Well, at least it will be virgin hair. I'll actually be able to see what my real color is after dying and streaking it all these years. That's something exciting to look forward to. But, today...the excitement is the mail.

I actually left the house today and drove the car myself to my doctor's appointment. It was thrilling. Seeing that I've been stuck in the house, even a doctor's appointment can be exciting. On Friday night, the office called to confirm and asked for "their favorite patient." I'm telling you, you have to train these doctor's offices. My mom is still in town, so she came with me. I had to restrain her from wanting to beat up the doctor since my right breast expander had to be removed. The doctor's appointment was with Dr. Plastic Surgeon. Luckily for the doctor, no beating occurred.

As soon as we got there, we were of course brought back immediately. My main reason for this appointment was to ask some questions. I can't have any surgeries until after chemotherapy in October, but he did say that I can have surgery as soon as two weeks after my last chemo, as long as my oncologist approves it. The scar on my right side looks like it's welded to my chest. I had to ask him if he was going to have to put his foot on my chest to pull apart the skin and muscle since it looked like it was cemented to my chest.

I was a bit concerned about that. He laughed and said no, it should not be a problem. I might only need the expander in for two weeks before I can have the new, exciting implants in. It will probably be an inpatient procedure so I can get extra IV antibiotics considering the last infection.

Nurse Hatchet drilled him about several things. I, of course, was sitting there like the medical spectacle I was to the two medical people sitting in front of me.

Good news! I'm healing properly and there should be no problems. Unfortunately for my husband, I won't be getting double F's in cup size. I will need at least two more surgeries on the breasts and then the oncologist and breast surgeon want the other female parts out. I think we'll get one thing done at a time. My goal is to have this behind me by the end of 2010 so that 2011 will start off with a new beginning.

We also asked for the operative reports on both surgeries. Everything looked like it was pretty straight forward. However, when he described me, he said, "The patient is a 39 year old female who looks her stated age." WHAT! I had to call the office and let them know that next time I prefer to be described as "Looks younger and cuter than stated age." I mean, really. I have to do mental status on people all the time and I would definitely describe myself as "Younger than stated age." I hope on the next operative report, I see the correction.

Dr. Plastic Surgeon asked if I had needed a prescription for a prosthesis to make me more symmetrical. I reminded him that he did already and I made the appointment with Cancer Center but had to cancel because I wasn't feeling well and never rescheduled. He seemed a bit shocked that I was walking around without at least a sock in my right side. I told him that, first of all, I hardly leave the house. If I really had some exciting event to go to I would probably shove a sock in my bra and put on my wig. But seeing that I'm not going to any red carpet events or even PTA meetings, I'm okay with not having "symmetry" for a couple of months. I think it would be different if I had hair.

If I had hair then the one breast look might look strange, but with no hair and no breast, I have all the necessary "Cancer Victim Walking" identifying marks. No sense hiding it. And again, I hardly leave the house with all of the symptoms and low white blood counts. Besides, at this point, I'm really not trying to impress anyone. I'm just excited if I can walk the aisles at Target and not get winded. Plus, with my current look, when I'm in any parking lot, people generally let me go past first. And, I don't even have to take off my hat to blind them with my baldness. If you thought I was pale before, you should see my head—again, about as white as you can get!

The other fun thing about having cancer is all of the medications you're on. Don't get me wrong. I love the medication. It's good and helps with the symptoms. It's picking it up at the pharmacy that is a bummer. Obviously, the pharmacist knows what the medications you're on are for, which is a bummer since it's a small town. I just loved it today when he said, "You want the Valium refilled also?" Of course, there were people around. I said, "Yeah, I really need it. My mother is still in town." (Just kidding, Mom.)

Glad I don't have anal cancer or anything like that. He might have said, "You need that anal cream refilled also?"

■

My mother left me to head back to Chicago last night. Okay, so it wasn't that dramatic; after all, she will be back in October for my final chemotherapy visit. But now I have no one to nag me about taking my medicine or eating on time or ask if I want a protein shake. Ah, I have to be a full-fledged adult again. Have you ever noticed once you're an adult, when your parents are around you tend to feel like you're 12 again? Given the past several months, I'm quite thankful that I have parents who are willing to jump on a plane to help out. I know a lot of other people are not as fortunate. Thanks, Mom!

This whole "being an adult" thing is not quite what the brochure promised. Remember when you were just dying to be an adult? You were going to keep all the lights on, stand in front of the refrigerator, not fold any towels, and no one was going to be there to tell you "no." Ah, those were the days. Now it's bills, taking care of your own kids and looking for the best insurance rates. Somehow not as glamorous as it seemed when we were younger. My seven-year old has already picked out a wife in his class. He said that he is going to get married and have a house. When I asked how he was going to pay for all of that he of course said, "Well, you and daddy." He has a long way to go, obviously.

This is the start of my "good week" before my fifth round of chemo on September 29th. I feel pretty good. I'm trying to focus on that because then I dread the feeling horrible after chemo. It feels really good to not get dizzy and have the chemo fog brain. Of course, even without hair, I have my blonde moments that I can't attribute to chemo. Interestingly, I like to play Scrabble. I usually have to beg either my husband or my mom to play with me. However, during my chemo fog phase, they ask me quite often to play! Taking advantage of a chemo patient like that!

I got a package in the mail the other day that was marked "To my favorite psychologist." Yet another sign of my adorableness. I'm sure that's what you were thinking. I immediately knew who it was from. This particular person sent me a hat that says "F#$& Cancer"—but the real "F" word and a t-shirt with "Cancer Sucks."

She said she thought it would be a good outfit to wear to my next chemo. I'm not sure if I can wear the hat, but maybe the shirt. I'm afraid my Lutheran guilt (you know, the sister of Catholic guilt) and upbringing in parochial schools for nine years of grammar school and four years of college (well, to be fair—college was not all what I would call religion based, if you know what I mean) will prevent me from wearing it. I'm sure if my former childhood pastors are reading this they will be proud of me. Although, that won't prevent me from wearing it around the house or on a day where I'm really crabby about the situation I'm in.

Also in the box was a pink rubber bracelet for breast cancer. I'm debating wearing that. This would definitely accessorize my current cancer victim look. Not to mention that it would readily explain to strangers—as if I really care what they think about me at this moment—what is going on with me. I have already received some pink ribbon pins and one that was bejeweled with pink crystals. I'm conflicted about wearing the outward "Breast Cancer" symbol at this point. I'm not sure if this is my little bit of denial or, dang it...maybe those pathology reports were wrong and someone is still going to call and say this was all a big mistake. Of course, that would mean I would have to get at least three different calls from three different pathologists. But hey, you never know.

I think it also means full acceptance of all of this. I'm sure many of you can relate to when you're going through something and a bit of denial creeps up every now and then and saves your sanity. All I have to do at this point is rub my bald head to know it's real. But there are some moments like today when I'm feeling good that I actually forget for a moment that I'm dealing with chemotherapy, blood counts, medications and surgeries. I will keep you updated on my bold decision to express myself outwardly. Don't get me wrong. I'm all for everyone else wearing their cause and I'm sure I will eventually, but not today.

Besides, have you noticed how many pink ribbons there are? They are everywhere! I was getting gas the other day and it was on the screen at the gas pump and then at the ATM and then on the laundry detergent and then on the cereal box and then on the advertisement at the mall and so on. It's everywhere! Which of course is a good thing but dang. Breast cancer research and awareness is great. It has come a long way and I'm benefiting from all of it. However, I can't help thinking how the evil oncologist I met with for a second opinion on chemotherapy said to me, "No one is ever going to do research on your type of cancer because less than one percent of breast cancer is the type you have." Again, not quite the pep talk I was expecting when I had the visit.

Ah, so since this is my good week I'm hoping to fill up on sugar and good stuff since my stomach and gut have calmed down. Unfortunately, no *Cake Boss* type cake this week, but those Oreos on the shelf are looking pretty good!

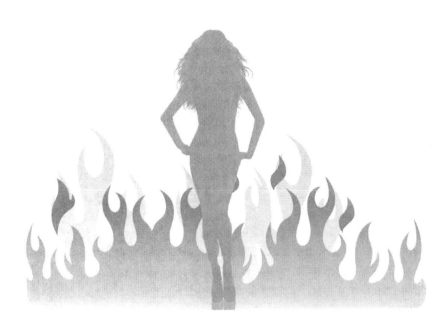

27 FIFTH CHEMO TREATMENT

September 26-October 3, 2010

I'm in "chemo wait" mode as Wednesday approaches. I have been feeling really good and have been trying to take advantage of it. It seems there's this fine balance between returning to normal activities and making sure I don't get sick. Also, one of our toilets was clogged and I worked on that, much to the horror of my mother. She noted that if I had a cut or anything on my hands it could easily get infected and would be very bad. Obviously I did the anti-bacterial wash down after that.

This is one of the reasons why I'm not supposed to get manicures during chemo. If I get a cuticle that is cut too closely and gets infected, I could be in trouble. I don't do my own nails very well, but I did finally paint my toes. Yes, I know, this is real excitement in my life. Chemo makes ridges in your nails that are oh-so-attractive but again, since I barely leave the house this does not seem to be an issue. Besides, who would really say to someone with no hair and one breast, "Boy, those nails look really unattractive!"

As I approach the end cycle of my chemotherapy, I keep thinking, "What comes next?"

I mean besides the surgeries. I know I have said this before, but it's hard to believe that I can't get some award or guarantee that the chemotherapy did its job. I almost feel like there should be some certificate of completion or diploma after finishing chemotherapy stating, "You're now free from cancer and have nothing to worry about for the rest of your life." I kind of doubt that they hand those out. But wouldn't that be nice? I was watching *Apollo 13* the other night because my son is into the rockets. They can put a man on the moon, but the human body and its diseases is still a mystery.

Then again, if I was living when they put a man on the moon, I probably wouldn't get the treatment I'm getting now. So I really shouldn't complain. And back then, they didn't have the fabulous pills they have now to help with the side effects of chemo.

This week will be a week of doctor's appointments again. Blood draws, chemo, shots, and fluids. Since I have no leisure skills, I did go online and was surfing the cancer websites again. I keep repeating this big mistake, and I blame my curiosity for it. I started to read the statistics and all of that good stuff. The research is always looking at "five year survival" rates. It really makes you think—what if you only had five years left? I think I would rather not know. Of course, there are the other sites, in case you missed them, about stenciling or essentially tattooing your bald head. One website even gave samples for essentially a "do it yourself" stencil. I don't know about you, but the thought of stenciling my head really does not sound appealing. I mean after all, what would one chose? Some of the stencils were flower patterns or puzzles. This would be really difficult for me, seeing that my entire wardrobe is either white t-shirts or solid colors. I have NO patterned clothing whatsoever, so why would I want that on my head?

Speaking of that, some of the cancer websites give other options for your bald head like wigs, hats and scarves. Again, all nice. I've been sporting a variety of solid color baseball caps. And yep, you guessed it, at least three of them are solid white. I had a suggestion that I should get one with rhinestones on it or a camouflage hat. Yeah. Not seeing that on my head, either. I suppose I could use this time in my life to suddenly be creative or more daring in how I dress. Like I mentioned before, the places that sell items for chemo patients are quite loud. Or as my brother would call some of my mother's more daring outfits, "old people camo." I guess I could try something. You know you have a bland wardrobe when your kids' bus driver says laughingly, "I didn't recognize you because you weren't wearing a white shirt." I know! I will live a little and get myself an off-white shirt!

As you can see, I really live on the edge.

■

I just completed my fifth chemotherapy treatment. Only one more to go! Before going to chemo, I found myself trying to decide what to wear. It's hot outside but for some reason, it always feels cold when you're getting the medications. I decided against wearing the "Cancer Sucks" shirt, so I went for a white t-shirt and my usual shorts. I have quite the chemo uniforms. I'm thinking about burning them when this is all done.

My adoring husband brought me to the chemo session. I actually got my iPad from the clutches of my daughter to try to play around with it.. I was in chemo ALL DAY. I started at 9am and didn't get out of the place until after 5pm. The reason is that they added a lot of extra medications and slowed down the Taxotere that seems to be most problematic. At one point, I had two IV lines running. I felt quite privileged.

As I mentioned, there has been a lot of staff turnover at the Cancer Center, but the new nurses really seem to know what they are doing. As a matter of fact, the nurse assigned to me told me that she had cancer at age 32 and had been through all of this already. And she had all her hair! She said she is about a five-year survivor and had to go through eight chemo treatments, radiation, and a lumpectomy! I guess after the first four treatments, they decided she needed four more because of her age. Wow. It was nice talking to someone who was younger than me and had been through the works already. She showed me a picture of her driver's license when her hair was just growing back in. Sometimes it really amazes me how many people are affected by breast cancer. I really had no idea.

Coming into chemo this time, the night before, my mom had dictated a nice long list to give to the PA. I'm sure he just loved that, but he did get everything done on the list. Since my blood counts were still low, I was able to get another shot to help with the anemia, so hopefully that will help with my recovery from yucky-ness during this treatment.

Today, you're actually getting the blow by blow of my getting fluids after chemo. I'm actually sitting in the Cancer Center getting a liter. Too bad it's not vodka or at least Ativan—no hangover with that stuff. Not my luck. But again, only one more treatment like this and then the surgeries start.

I'm really hoping to leave all of this behind me in 2011 and get back to normalcy—whatever that might look like after breast cancer. I think the big issue after that will be getting my hair back. Like I said before, it takes a while for it to come back, but I'm getting used to not having hair. However, think about how much hair has to do with our self-image. I was watching the new television show *Running Wilde,* with Keri Russell. Remember when she was in *Felicity* and she cut her hair before filming and the ratings plummeted? The director of the studio demanded that no one cut their hair without his permission.

Other than that, things are going pretty well. I feel good today. This is good because for the last two treatments, I started feeling awful the night of chemo, so I think this is an improvement. Maybe all of the extra drugs they gave me this time will help with that. We love drugs. I was reading how before the good anti-nausea medication, about 50 percent of patients would drop out of chemotherapy because it was too difficult. I'm lucky that I'm able to have the drugs—even if they are $100 a pill!

■

When Saturday hit, so did the body aches. I received two injections on Thursday, one for anemia and one to improve the white blood cells in my body. That second one really gives bone pains and aches. This time I got hit hard with it. Chemo brain seems to be worsening for me as well, and the pain I suffer seems to only further induce my inability to focus. I cannot concentrate on anything more intense than episodes of *Everybody Loves Raymond.* This is actually pretty sad because I believe I have seen all of them—that was part of my seclusion after having my son.

The good news, which my husband keeps reminding me, is that I only have one more to go. I'm quite sure that after this last chemo treatment and fluids that my head looked pretty much like "Jack" in the Jack in the Box commercials. I woke up Saturday morning and literally had slits where my eyes used to be. Just call me Big Head. I think I had to loosen my hat a little bit. Even my fingers were swollen. So I had chubby fingers with nails that have ridges on them.

The other thing I keep forgetting about chemo is that it essentially burns out your taste buds for a couple of weeks. Before chemo, I can actually taste food, particularly chocolate. However, my taste buds are burned again and everything tastes like cardboard. Even water doesn't taste very satisfying. My babysitter had a birthday this week and I got her a chocolate cake. That didn't even taste good, plus it hurt my stomach! This chemo thing is really forcing me to eat healthier...or blander.

But, as long as all goes well, my last chemo should be on October 20th. I have an appointment with my oncologist this week and bloodwork. It has been a slow week at the cancer office! I'm anticipating that my WBC is going to be super low this time again and I'll be stuck in the house. Before chemo, my WBC was only 3.8, when normal is 4. Last chemo, I was up closer to the 10 range. We'll see; maybe the miracle shots will help all of that. You'd think they could come up with a miracle shot to grow hair back faster.

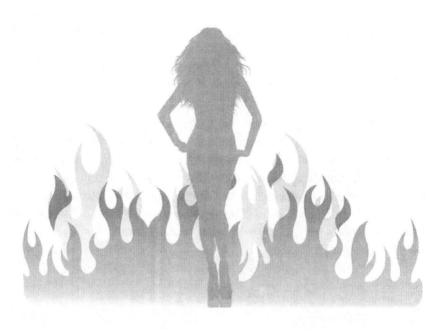

28 BREAST CANCER AWARENESS MONTH

October 7-11, 2010

Yesterday, I had another checkup with the oncologist. These checkups really seem to be more like cheerleading sessions. Dr. Perky told me that I'm doing great and to hang on because there is only one more left. She's so positive and perky—even more so than me, and I thought that was hard to do. Of course, my level of perkiness has been quite lowered by all of the chemo medications, so I have an excuse.

I couldn't help but feel like a science experiment because she had her PA in the room again. Yes, part of his job was to take notes so she didn't have to, but I noticed that when I walked into the room, the PA was not with her during her consult before me. As the appointment went along, I realized part of the reason is possibly because I'm the anomaly in the practice, even though Dr. Perky denies it. Metaplastic cancer is less than one percent of all breast cancers.

The PA is always asking questions like, "Do you see that a lot?" when referring to something specific about my type of cancer. In a way, I should feel good because I'm the center of attention. Appointments like this make me think that I'm glad I didn't go to a university or clinic setting. I would probably just be treated like a number instead of favorite patient status. Academics generally don't have a sense of humor, as I have painfully found out.

Dr. Perky also let me know the chemo fog that I've been having lately, compounded by the Ambien I'm taking for sleep, will probably worsen over the next several weeks with my last treatment. Somehow she has a way of delivering not so great news in an upbeat matter. So, when she says these things, I get distracted by the perkiness and don't really think about it until on the way home. She said something about doing crossword puzzles and stuff like that to improve my cognition after my last chemotherapy. Crossword puzzles! I got into the car and thought to myself, "Did I just get a prescription for crossword puzzles?" Really? I hate crossword puzzles. I might have to actually use the book I bought my parents the last time they were here called "Senior Moments" with cognition improvement exercises. I'm pretty sure that I will be able to get up to speed after chemo, but right now I feel scattered. But again, I'm blonde (when I have hair), so that could be impacting things as well.

Speaking of forgetting, I finally remembered to ask Dr. Perky about the rationale behind my chemotherapy protocol. Of course, I could have asked this before but I always forget. When I first met with her back in May, she said that I would only be getting four cycles of two chemotherapy medications. When I showed up for the first chemo appointment, I was told I would be getting six cycles of three medications including the Taxotere, which is the one that wreaks the havoc on my body. I asked her what happened at the tumor board to change her mind.

Apparently, because of the rarity of the cancer and my age, she was told to "throw everything at me" and treat the cancer like it's a triple negative cancer—meaning the estrogen, progesterone and HER2 receptors are all negative. This is also a rare cancer. However, my progesterone receptor is positive.

Of course, I have to have the weird cancer. Because of this, I will most likely have to take some other type of medication after chemotherapy which will lower my odds of recurrence. In her perky voice, she mentioned that since we now know that my body can make cancer, we want to lower my risks. She also said that, about three weeks after chemotherapy ends, she wants a PET scan done to assure me that they got everything. So again, Dr. Perky sends mixed messages. Why doesn't medication come with a guarantee?! I wonder how often I can get a PET scan. If I was some celebrity, maybe I would have one installed in my house. Kind of like how Jenny McCarthy had an oxygen chamber installed in her house for her son's autism.

■

It's Breast Cancer Awareness Month, and there's pink everywhere. I was at the grocery store yesterday and all of the cashiers had on pink aprons. When I'm really focused on something—which is hard these days with chemo brain—I forget what I'm going through. Unless I look in the mirror, I sometimes I just forget. Forgetting is a way of coping, after all.

But this month, as soon as I leave the house, there are pink ribbons everywhere. I don't know that I'm ready to wear pink all over. I saw a picture in the newspaper this morning of one woman at a Susan B. Komen event wearing a hot pink wig along with a sparkly survivor banner across her chest and a pink tiara. Yeah. I'm just not seeing that happening with me. When I checked out at the grocery store, the clerk asked me if I wanted to donate a dollar to breast cancer. Of course, I had to laugh because she wasn't able to look me in the eye when she asked. I smiled and said, "I gave at the office."

I'm considering wearing the pink bracelet when I have to go out this month. But I haven't decided yet. I kind of figure that I'm a walking billboard for breast cancer at this point. Maybe I will just wear my plain pink hat. Now that I think about it, probably the best time to wear it will be after I have my reconstruction surgery and actually have two breasts again. At that point, my hair will just be starting—hopefully—to grow back in. At least the bracelet might explain the lack of hair or the shockingly short hair I will be sporting. Without the bracelet, someone might think I'm jealous of Portia's relationship with Ellen DeGeneres. I'm a little worried about that. The baldness makes a statement. Short, spikey hair sometimes makes another statement that I don't want to send. I might actually take the wig out at that point.

I have to say, I'm feeling very good today. I think the extra shots for anemia are really helping. I feel like I'm getting back to my old self. I even painted my nails! On my own of course—real manicures aren't allowed. At least the polish covers the ridges in my nails. It dawned on me today that I really only have one treatment left. That means only one more time feeling lousy. I mean, it'll still take a while until I'm back up to my usual hyper self, but really only one more time feeling horrible.

I have surgeries afterward, but recovering from a surgery compared to the systemic illnesses that chemotherapy causes seems almost minor at this point. And, of course, I will have good drugs after surgery for pain. My fatigue is not as bad as it was and most of my gut issues this round of chemo were immediately following the treatment. This really got me excited. I have had a couple of people ask how I'm going to celebrate my last chemo. I think that I'm not going to do a whole lot of celebrating until all the surgeries are over. After all, right after surgery I feel like crap, and who wants to celebrate when you feel like that? I will celebrate in spirit.

I'm excited, but I don't think that I'm going to be drenched in pink or watch every episode of Showtime's new series, *The Big C*. I think I'm cancer-ed out for a while. I still have to watch what I eat, which is definitely a reminder. I used to have a stomach of steel, meaning I could eat chocolate, mildly spicy foods, and BBQ sauce. Now, I have to watch all of that lest I get sick. My husband had some BBQ beef the other night and I could hardly stand the smell of it. Hopefully, that will all go away also after chemotherapy.

In the meantime, I'm enjoying just feeling better. I'm still in the house most of the time, but somehow it doesn't seem to matter as much as I thought it would in the beginning. I sometimes have the urge to flash someone on the side where I don't have a breast and just a scar. I mean, technically it's not flashing if there's no breast there, right?

I guess that would still be inappropriate behavior, though. I would rather do something like that when my mother is here and we're out in public together and then I can yell, "I'm her daughter!" just to mortify her. I'll have to think about that. Besides, I think by now the people at Target and the McDonald's drive-thru (which are basically the only places I go to) know who I am. I've become the regular character.

I actually might be well enough to make my kids' parent/teacher conferences this week! That is a huge step, since I haven't set foot in the school since they started this year. Who would have thought that would be the highlight of my week? How things change.

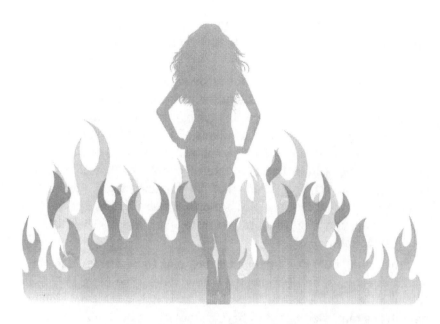

29 LAST CHEMO TREATMENT
October 19-24, 2010

Tomorrow is my last and final chemotherapy! However, both of the kids came down with head colds and, of course, I had to get it. Luckily, I didn't get it when my white blood count was really low. I lost my voice earlier in the week and am still not feeling 100%. I don't have a fever and I didn't get a call from the Cancer Center saying that I can't have chemo tomorrow. I'm really excited, seeing that this means that this long journey is finally winding down.

Although I have had this bad head cold, it didn't completely wipe me out because I'm still getting the shot that helps with anemia. I have a lot more energy and don't feel like a zombie. It's also a bonus that when I stand up I don't get dizzy. My taste buds are still shot but they will come back with time, and my stomach is still pretty sensitive. I had Burger King burger the other day and that didn't end well.

I also had a great visit from a friend and her niece this weekend. I'm proud to say that I only had to take a nap once! And I was able to walk the mall without having to sit down or be carried out due to exhaustion or dizziness! The milestones! The things you take for granted when you're healthy! Of course, we were at the Disney store and a woman who worked there who had really short hair said to me, "I wore hats all the time instead of wigs. I only just started going without a hat." She was really nice. I then mentioned that this week was my last chemotherapy appointment and then she says, "Oh, that was my worst one!" Great, I didn't need to hear that. I said that I'm excited it's the last one. The last time being really sick. The last time, could it be true?

My mom is flying in late tonight because she wanted to be there for the last chemo. Of course, we'll have to bring the staff some snacks. I'll still be monitored closely for a long time, and I think the oncologist wants to have that PET scan done in a couple of weeks to assure they got everything. I'm pretty confident they did.

I've been trying to keep myself busy since I've been feeling better. I've actually left the house and went to lunch with a new friend! Over the weekend, my husband had a party with his poker friends for my birthday and one of the women who plays poker. I was offered several shots but, of course, could not partake in any of the activities. I still get to bed pretty early. And, since my friend was in, we stayed up talking. That was probably the latest I have stayed up in months.

I had to hit the pharmacy and get all of my chemo drugs (again, hopefully for the last time!) and spend the big dollar on the three little pills that are going to magically take away my nausea from the chemo. Someone asked me if all of my research I did in the beginning helped me to get through all of this. My first response, was "Well, studies indicate if you have a good attitude about it, you're going to do much better." But then I was completely honest and said, "It's the good drugs." If it wasn't for the drugs they have now, I don't know that I would have made it this far.

If I had to sit next to the porcelain god for months at a time, I don't know that I could be that perky either about getting chemo. I'm not sure how those people, who I encounter in private practice, tell me they "don't believe in medications." I bet they would be singing a different song altogether!

There was an article in *People*—or as I like to call it "the news"— about a reporter who had triple negative breast cancer. They showed her post-treatment with her new short hairstyle. It came in dark and gray! I'm not looking forward to that. I can't complain. She found an eight-centimeter tumor and had to have a lot more chemotherapy than

I did. She found it when she was breastfeeding her last child and they didn't do anything about it until months later, so it grew. Just goes to show—if you feel something that's not right, listen to your gut and go in and have it checked out. Don't wait around!

I have saved every card and cherished every voicemail and email I've received from people along the way. Never underestimate the power of a kind word or a simple email that says, "I was thinking about you." Some days, those simple little things have helped me get through the day.

Although Wednesday was my last chemo treatment, I've had chemo brain since then. When Dr. Perky said this was going to be the hard one, she was right. I've been in bed since then. Literally. No television. No reading. Nothing. My entire body has ached and I've been sick to my stomach, but at least it was the last one.

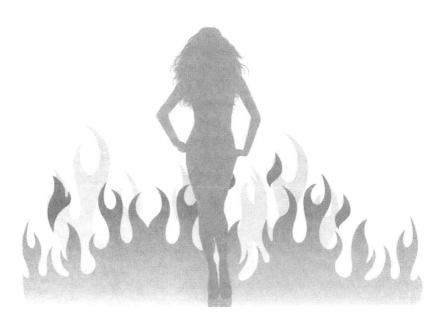

30 NO MORE CHEMO!
November 4-8, 2010

Yesterday, I had my appointment with the oncologist, Dr. Perky, and it looks like my chemotherapy is behind me! This, of course, will depend on next week's PET scan, but she's confident we won't find anything because the cancer was caught so early! The thrill! The excitement!

The chemo will still be in my body for several more weeks, but at least it's over. She did give me an antibiotic for my head cold that has lasted for over three weeks now. Of course, it was an expensive one that is not covered by my insurance, but still—it already seems to be working! The staff kind of freaked out when taking my vitals because I had a low-grade fever.

Since my last update and the conversation with first OB/GYN, I've been trying not to focus on the fact that reoccurrence is a possibility with this type of cancer. As a result, my type-A self went back to the research—bad idea. The research still indicates that metaplastic cancer is not good. However, trying to look at things objectively—which is very difficult at this stage—most of the women in those studies didn't get treatment until their tumors were significantly larger than mine. Coming into the appointment with Dr. Perky, I had a list of questions prepared to address these concerns.

I was in the waiting room yesterday and started talking to a woman who I thought was there with someone getting chemo. Turns out she had breast cancer 10 years ago and then it came back in her lymph nodes a few years ago. She found both the lumps herself. She was on a check-up visit with Dr. Perky. She explained to me how she has already had two rounds of chemo. The first round was without the revolutionary new anti-nausea medications that they have now. She said the second round was a world of difference. I was very encouraged by that, but even more so that she now had a full head of hair—short hair—but hair nonetheless. Funny how when you don't have hair, suddenly hairstyles really start to interest you! As she got up to go to her appointment with Dr. Perky, I was left to sit there for about an hour—she was running way behind. For a moment, my mind started racing about reoccurrence. The type of cancer I have usually comes back in the bones and lungs, not the lymph nodes, meaning that I won't necessarily be able to feel a lump. Instead of freaking myself out about that, I instead turned to a mindless fashion magazine with Courtney Cox on the cover, looking at how they airbrushed all of her wrinkles out. Too bad cancer can't be airbrushed.

Dr. Perky came and got me and I had my questions in hand. The thing about Dr. Perky is that as confrontational (which for me is not very confrontational) as I try to be, she's so disarming. She's so sincere and caring and so damn perky. The first thing she asked me was how I felt my rapport was with the OB/GYN consult I had. I thought that was a brilliant way to start. I told her I didn't really care for her because instead of talking about how two different specialists are recommending that my ovaries come out, she gave me a lecture on the problems of early menopause. At this point, seeing that I didn't care for this doctor, Dr. Perky gave her opinion, which was that she didn't send me there for Dr. Gyn's opinion, she sent me there for surgery.

She went on to say that many of the GYNs don't get the connection between the ovaries and cancer. How good was that? She strategically waited to see what I thought about the doctor first. I just love that—sorry, the psychologist in me never seems to stop working. Anyway, I told her that I already have another appointment scheduled with the GYN that my breast surgeon recommended. She knew who that doctor was right away and said that she was very good and that I "will just love her." Of course, it made me think, "Why didn't you recommend her in the first place?" But then I remembered her PA had recommended the first GYN.

Given Dr. Perky's opinion of the first GYN and her conversation with her, it sounds like she had to convince her why my ovaries should come out. It made me think that she probably had to over stress the notion that reoccurrence of cancer is likely to get her point across. I was able to breathe a sigh of relief—for a moment. I then went on to question her about the PET scan scheduled for next week. What happens if they find something? Then what? Should I be getting emotionally prepared for that? She told me not to worry, that they've done every aggressive thing they can and won't find anything. Okay. I can deal with that, but then I had to ask, "But if they do find something, do YOU call me directly, or will it be one of the MAs?" She smiled and said that she would call me and have me come back to the office. You know it's bad news when the doctor actually calls you directly, so I wanted to be prepared. But again, she's sure she won't find anything. Cross your fingers.

In the meantime, she has cleared me to move forward with my surgeries. She said that the 10 day antibiotic I'm taking should clear everything up and that I can move forward. Because I'm going to have so many surgeries, she does not want to draw the tumor markers until after the first of the year because any inflammation from the surgeries could give a false positive. The tumor markers will be compared to the first ones I had drawn before I started with chemotherapy and surgeries. These will continue to be drawn for a while to monitor if the cancer is comes back.

She also said my port can come out! The port is the annoying thing now sticking out on my chest where they'd administered all of the chemotherapy. This is great news because during my last round of chemo, there were about three people who came in to have theirs flushed. If you keep the port, it usually means more chemo and it has to be flushed once a month! Of course, it will leave a battle scar, but right now, my chest looks like a bad road map of the Himalayas anyway, so I'm not going to fret about that.

Another bonus is that because my ovaries will be coming out, Dr. Perky does not feel that I need to be on any long-term medications! I'm sure this will be reviewed on an ongoing basis, but that's great news! Again, she noted that by the end of this we'll have done pretty much everything possible to prevent reoccurrence—the mastectomy, chemotherapy, the ovaries—when some other people might have just gone with the lumpectomy (of course, if I did that, I would be worrying about finding another lump and wouldn't be getting the added bonus of new perky boobs!).

At the end of the appointment, Dr. Perky said I had to come in next week for labs again, but then I didn't need to see her until early February unless something comes up. WHAT? I said, "Are you sure? That's it?" It almost felt like a letdown. "You mean I only have to deal with the surgeons for the next couple of months?" She said that yes, that's correct. I half expected a parade and confetti when I left the exam room that I had completed my sometimes four visits a week to the oncologist. But guess what?! There was no confetti. No parade. No one cheering as I left! I was almost in tears because I was so happy, but then again, when you have your entire body monitored so closely for so long it almost feels like, "Wait, you're sending me off into the jungle all by myself?"

She assured me that I will have to see her religiously every three months for the next two years. I will have occasional scans, and if I get any symptoms, I will need to come back. At that moment, I realized why she kept asking me throughout this what was I going to do to celebrate. This whole time I was thinking that I didn't need that, but now I see why some people do have a celebration. Of course, in my head, this still isn't done until the surgeries are over, but somehow not seeing the oncologist every week feels like a safety net was just dropped. So, I just might do something celebratory in the future. Seeing that this good old German-Irish girl hasn't had a drink since the day before my surgery—it will undoubtedly involve something fruity with a little umbrella. I will save some of my anti-nausea medication for the day after.

Not only that, but I really felt like since chemotherapy was over, somehow I should have walked out of the office with a full head of hair—but that didn't happen either. Dang. I have to wait for it to grow out, which won't even start to happen for a couple of weeks. But again, on the bright side, chemotherapy is over with! No more expensive drugs. No more sitting in the office for a whole day, getting drugs that you know will only make you sick for the next week or more. No more anticipating the next chemotherapy and how it will affect your entire system.

As I walked out to my car, there was no celebration except in my head. One major milestone is behind me. Of course, this won't be officially confirmed until the PET scan results come back, but I'm going to cherish this moment for a while.

In the meantime, I received more good news. I contacted the plastic surgeon's office, where surely I'm the most adorable patient they've ever had, and asked for them to start looking into scheduling surgery to get my expander replaced, if possible, before Thanksgiving. I have an appointment with the doctor on Monday, but Nurse Hatchet recommended that I call ahead of time because they'll have to coordinate with the breast surgeon for the port removal. My secret insider at the plastic surgeon's office texted me that I'm on the schedule for Friday, November 19th for the afternoon! I will be having the surgery at the hospital in case I have to stay overnight. If you recall when I had the expanders in the first time, it was quite painful and I had to stay extra days. I'm hoping this will not be the case, but better to be on the safe side with the happy drugs they give you in the hospital than at home suffering.

My hope is that I can have the expanders removed a few weeks later and have the ovaries out all in December! And then: Welcome 2011! I can see the light at the end of the tunnel!

■

This weekend I had my first adventure out of the house wearing my wig. I had to meet with a potential business referral for when I'm well. I decided to go with the wig and stuff a sock in my bra to see how it went. First of all, I felt like a complete old lady wearing the wig. I'm not sure why, since a lot of young people wear wigs and hair extensions. I don't know if it's the color or the style, but it felt weird. Maybe I really need a longer one so that I can swing my hair around and feel more stripper-like. The one I have feels kind of soccer mom-ish. Thank goodness it wasn't that hot out this weekend, or I would have been itching up a storm. I even wore jewelry and real shoes—flip-flops and gym shoes have pretty much been my wardrobe. The wig thing is weird because it has bangs. I ended up pulling up some pictures of myself taken before chemo and I really miss my hair.

Before I left, I asked my son how I looked. He told me I looked okay, but I'll have nice long hair by the time Christmas comes. Yeah, that isn't going to happen, but maybe the wishful thinking of a child can make my hair grow longer and faster than normal.

Interestingly, once I met with the person, we started talking and it turned out that she had just been diagnosed with thyroid cancer two days earlier. So, I let her in on my secret and then asked her if she could tell it was a wig. She said "no" very sincerely, so I think I actually believe her! Still, I think I might have a friend of mine, who loves wigs and hair, take me out to get a new wig. I definitely think I'm going to look into extensions once I get some growth coming back.

Over the weekend, this one appointment completely wore me out. I think it was the combination of actually sitting up with a live person doing work and the emotional toll of wondering, "Can they tell I'm wearing a wig or not?" Somehow since chemo is over, I feel like I should be back to my old self, but I'm still easily fatigued and, unfortunately, still have a bit of a cold. The antibiotics have helped tremendously, but my stamina is very low. In my head, I should be off and running already, but my body is telling me a different story.

Anyway, I'm glad I can wear the wig out again without feeling completely weird. After all, it was a $400 item. Who knew fake hair was so much money? You can bet that in a couple of weeks that price will pale in comparison to the hair growth products I'll be buying once my hair does start to bud! I'm actually quite comfortable with the hat over my bald head. However, since I'm a psychologist, once I do start seeing patients again, I don't want the patient to feel like they can't tell me their problems because I look like I'm sick or have more problems than they do. Never a good combination for therapy.

I hope I didn't freak out anybody who might have seen me take off my wig once I got in my car. On the other hand, at this point, in terms of regular people—meaning not patients—I really don't care what other people think—one of the many blessings that have come out of this experience. You don't like me or how I do things? So what? I'm beating cancer. Petty people don't really matter anymore. Not that they did before, really. I like to think of myself as a very confident person, anyway. But an experience like this really highlights what's important— and really, hair is overrated.

This morning I'm off to the plastic surgeon for my pre-operative appointment. Surgery is scheduled for November 19, 2010 to have the right expander put in and the port taken out! The end is near! Thursday is the PET scan. I hope they don't find that my brain has shrunk with the chemo! Some days that's exactly how I feel.

■

I went to the plastic surgeon's office on Monday. The office manager/MA came in the room first to go over all of the pre-operative information, including risks and complications. Somehow I don't remember anyone doing this for me the first time. She went over how I can't lift anything for a while. No vigorous exercise of any kind for six weeks (like I've been doing any of that lately). Ugh! It just reminded me of how painful the first surgery was.

Dr. Plastic Surgeon came in and slid his chair far away from me and said with a smile, "I doubt it will hurt like last time, but I'm going to say that from here so you don't hit me." At least he's gotten to know me. We'll see how the surgery goes. I had in my mind that it wasn't going to be as big as a deal as the chemo symptoms, but then they have to go over all of the risks, complications, and what to expect. This includes that I'm to come to the hospital with no makeup! Again! I better get a Sharpie marker and write my name on my limbs because without makeup and hair, I'm virtually unrecognizable. I want to make sure they operate on the correct person. The other thing I was thinking about was, what if he puts the expander in upside down? I wonder if that makes a difference. Yes, I know. I'm just looking for trouble at this point.

I'm definitely bored of this whole being sick thing. I'm over it. The problem is, my body isn't over it yet.

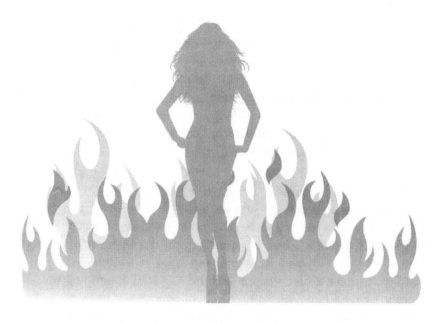

31 PET SCAN & POST-CHEMO

November 12-15, 2010

This morning, I actually feel a little better after getting a lot of rest. Go figure; the human body heals better when it's not trying so hard.

Yesterday, I had my post-chemo PET scan at 7am. This is the PET scan that was to determine if I had any more cancer or if it had spread. So needless to say I was quite nervous. With the rarity of my cancer type and the needed expert opinion that my doctor had solicited, the results of the PET scan could possibly determine the rest of my life. That probably accounted for part of the Debbie Downer mood—that and hearing all of the risks and complications of my upcoming surgery next week. In addition, I had to be on a high-protein, low-sugar, low-carb diet for 48 hours before surgery.

Now, I know perfectly well how to do that since I do weight loss surgery evaluations for a living. But when you're crabby and in a Debbie Downer mood and not able to have chocolate, it certainly adds to the irritation. Of course, during this 48-hour period, I think I came across every piece of sugar and chocolate in the house. The cancer supposedly processes sugar differently, which is why I can't have it prior to the PET scan. Too much sugar beforehand can give false positives. So, like a little soldier, I stuck to the diet.

I arrived at the imaging center and guess who's there? One of the women I saw every week for chemo and her partner. I didn't exactly bond with this couple when I was there, but there they were, waving to me as I walked in like I was a long-lost friend. So much for anonymity. The same technician was there to take me back for the PET scan. I have to be juiced up with a radioactive isotope for 45 minutes prior. It comes in a huge metal syringe that looks like it came from a 1950's sci-fi movie. No, I didn't glow afterward, but I sure felt like I was going to.

After the injection, they have you sit in a room with a supposedly calm video called *The Blue Planet*, which is about ocean life. At first you think it's going to be calm, and then you see whales and birds eating up other creatures. Not calming at all. I pulled out my Kindle and tried to read some of my positive thinking literature. Of course, the chapter I start out reading is all about how a positive attitude has proven to help with illness and improve the immune system. Of course, I know all of this. I preach it to others but it's sometimes hard to follow all the time.

After the 45 minutes are over, I get to sit in a big tube for about 40 minutes as each part of my body is scanned. The technician does a test run to make sure I fit—I did, with plenty of room, thank you—and to make sure I don't freak out from being confined. Having these tests always reminds me of the scene in *The Incredibles* when Mr. Incredible is on the island and completely out of shape and they try to shoot him out of a tube. Thankfully, that was not the case with me.

I have to lay completely still for all of that time with my hands above my head. I used my breathing and meditation techniques that I often teach patients. It worked like a charm for those of you who "don't believe in that psychology crap." When I was done, I boldly asked the technician this time if he saw anything. It was fun to see him squirm, because he isn't supposed to say anything. He said, "Oh, you don't want my opinion. You want the guy who has 15 years of school behind him telling you." I replied that I was sure he knew what he was doing since he did it all day. He did mention that usually after chemo, your body is completely rebuilding, so often the PET scans look a little different. Another reminder of why I probably feel like crap.

My body is completely rebuilding itself after the abuse it took from the chemo. After using my psychological power skills, he let me look at the scan on the computer. It was actually pretty cool to see your insides rotating around 360 degrees. He pointed out my liver and kidneys. You could also see my one expander and the outline of my body. I have to say that I looked quite good on the PET scan. The chemo diet—which I don't recommend—has made me lose a couple of those pesky unwanted pounds. Of course, just because my outline on a PET scan looked decent doesn't mean that translates to a bikini-ready body. It was nice to see the images but, of course, I really didn't know what I was looking for and wouldn't know if my body was riddled with cancer. However, I didn't see anything out of the ordinary. As I left, the technician said I should know the results in a day or two, Monday at the latest. More waiting.

When I got home, I went right to bed. I decided I would rest again. I'm constantly shocked at how much these appointments take it out of me. And, of course, I went right for something sugary and chocolaty. Ah, it was wonderful. Surprisingly, about two hours after I got home, my oncologist's office called to tell me that the PET scan was completely clear! There was no cancer and no unusual uptake to be concerned about. That means the cancer is gone! That suspicious spot on my chest wall they saw in the first PET scan was probably nothing. That's just fabulous news! The cancer is gone. The last six to seven months, and now until the end of the year, have all been worth it...even if I have no hair and no energy.

Now my job is to make sure I'm completely well for the surgery next week. Although I'm not looking forward to surgeries, at least I know that the light at the end of the tunnel is near. One day I will have my energy back and be my usual perky self with perky breasts! It'll be nice to reconnect with the rest of the world and all of my friends and family who have been so supportive through all of this. So, again, I will be resting today and not pushing myself so hard like I usually do. I suppose that I'm going to learn many lessons from this whole experience.

■

I'm done with chemo! However, little did I know that some of the side effects will keep on going for a while. I spent most of the weekend with body and muscle aches. Sunday, it was really bad. I almost thought I had the flu. After a little research, I found out that this is a common occurrence and some patients continue to have these aches following Taxotere for up to a year or more!

I'm glad I didn't get any of the neuropathy that can happen in your extremities. Apparently that takes a very long time to go away. I thought for sure I was going crazy yesterday. I wasn't sure if it was the flu, so I didn't want to exercise and make it worse. As a result, I might be moving around like an old lady for a while. At least I'm cancer-free, so I'm trying not to complain, but it does take a little longer to get out of bed these days.

I've also been researching how I should eat after cancer treatment. Obviously healthy eating and exercising are going to be important. My main exercise is walking or doing the treadmill. However, the healthy eating... well... Most research says that your main diet should consist of 80 percent fruits and vegetables. Eighty percent! I don't know how I'm going to do that. If it was 80 percent cheese I might be able to do that, but fruits and vegetables?! That is a category of the food pyramid that I usually avoid. I like to save my calories for things like chocolate. Studies also show that you need to avoid sugar as well and caffeine! I hope I don't have to turn into a hippie vegan! I don't have the hair for it right now first of all. Second of all, most of my wardrobe is white t-shirts— not tie-dyes. I rarely even hit Jamba Juice or places like that.

I suppose I'll be my own worst patient when it comes to healthy eating. Don't get me wrong. I love certain things like watermelon and broccoli. The problem is, most fruits and vegetables require some work—other than pushing buttons on a microwave—which I excel at, by the way. Most of them require cutting and chopping, putting them in containers. I walk by the melons and the pineapples in the grocery store because of the work they entail just to eat them. As a matter of fact, I don't think that I even know how to cut a pineapple.

Wait. I just thought of a great solution! Wine is made of grapes! I can get my fruits that way! And Bloody Marys are made with tomato juice— there are my vegetables! Of course, I will have to acquire a taste for those. Strawberry and banana daiquiris! The possibilities are endless!

Unfortunately for me, I found that post-cancer, one needs to limit alcohol as well because it's pure sugar. Well, maybe I can do a mind-over-matter thing and tell myself that the wine is filled with cancer-fighting components. Or just exercise more.

There's so much to think about after getting cancer. Of course I don't want it to come back, but I don't want to be a celery-chewing, wheat grass-eating cow afterward. I suppose I can stock up on the vegetables that come in the self-steaming bag and utilize my microwaving skills!

This week, I'm in waiting mode again as I wait for my first surgery on Friday. I sent my latest bloodwork and PET scan results to my plastic surgeon. I told him that I was cancer-free, so all he has to do now is make his favorite patient—who looks much younger and cuter than stated age—now look fabulous.

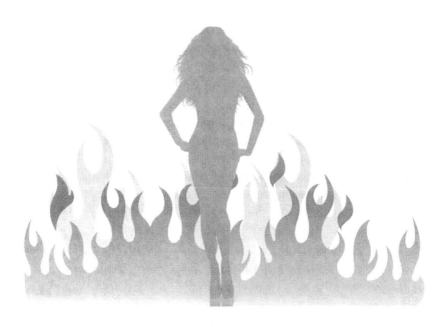

32 ANOTHER SURGERY
November 17-24, 2010

My first surgery is on Friday. I'm having my right expander put back in; hopefully it will not be as painful as the last time. They moved the time from 11am to 1:30pm (meaning that I'll be without food for basically most of the day), so I'm sure that you'll be happy that you won't be around me. It won't be pretty. The hospital called and told me that I have to take two showers with some special soap. They didn't ask me to do that last time. Am I dirtier this time? Don't they essentially hose you down with the iodine stuff anyway before surgery? They have the operating room scheduled for at least two hours, but the nurse said that I'll be in recovery for a minimum of one hour. I hope that's enough time to get the good drugs.

One thing I have learned through all of this—make sure you befriend the anesthesiologist. If you don't, you might not come off the anesthesia happy. They're also responsible for all of the drugs you're given while in pre-op and post-op. I personally like the shot that totally removes the memory of when I went under. I always make sure that I chat it up with the anesthesiologist before going under. I make sure that they are not going to be playing Scrabble on their phone or calling their girlfriend when they are supposed to be monitoring my vitals. I basically use my psychological powers of guilting them into top performance. I've worked at surgery centers and have seen some anesthesiologists multitask when they should be watching the patient. Too much information isn't always good, eh?

I've been working on other solutions to my 80 percent post-cancer fruit and vegetable diet. For example, how about fruit roll ups? I wonder if they count. Or Kellogg's makes a very good "fruit crisp" breakfast bar. What about chocolate covered fruit? That might be a good alternative as well. Dress up cauliflower with cheese? What about strawberry cheesecake? I'm pretty sure that the research probably means that they want actual unadulterated fruits and vegetables, but of course they didn't specify. I have resolved myself to explore this loophole.

At least from what I recall, I still do have some chemo brain going on. So far, I'm not doing too well at this, but I figure that I have until the end of the year to get myself ready. After all, my appetite and gut still are not that great. I keep thinking my body should be fine, but last night, I thought that I'd be up all night with intestinal cramps. Spicy food is still not a good thing right now. My brain keeps thinking that I'm doing better than I am. Again, I'm faced with the dilemma between my mind and my body, a conflict instigated by cancer. With both acting rather stubbornly, it's seemingly difficult that they will ever reach a consensus.

The hair update—no growth yet. Nothing. Nada. As a matter of fact, I think I have lost more from my eyebrows in the last couple of weeks than I have in the whole chemo period. At least it will eventually grow back. I'm getting so accustomed to being bald that I've walked out of the house a couple of times without my hat, much to the shock of the kids' bus driver. He asked me if I was trying to tan the old noggin.

At least in a couple of days, my chest will be even, so I won't look totally malformed and bald. These are the exciting things in my life these days. Aren't you jealous? Cancer is a bitch no matter how you slice it, but a positive attitude does help. Thank God that all of my preaching to patients all these years actually is sinking into my own head. I guess in retrospect, I should have done a study on myself when this first started. I was pretty mental at the beginning, like most people who are just told they have an aggressive form of cancer. Not a good time to start a study on yourself.

Well, I'll keep you updated on how the surgery goes. Hopefully it'll be unremarkable and a very boring story. Wouldn't that be nice?

■

Everything went well. The hospital where the surgery was held was a little confusing. Last time I had surgery, I was admitted through the emergency room, so we parked over there. Turns out the front of the hospital is on the complete opposite side of the building. When we got in the building, we asked a couple of ladies for whom obviously English was a second language. They escorted us right up to the actual surgery wing.

Once we finally got to admitting, they took me right away. My paperwork said "stat" on it because they were trying to all get home for the afternoon. Or at least, that was my assumption. Interestingly, the woman who registered me had my same plastic surgeon and went on and on and on about how wonderful he is and what a great job he did with her reconstructive surgery. Since I'd had surgery there before, I only had to sign a couple of pages and I was off. She escorted me up to the surgery wing—where we'd been originally. The room was full of people. Apparently, this was also the waiting room for ICU patients, so there were some sad-looking folks.

Almost immediately, I got called back to start the pre-op procedures. I had to have blood drawn. They missed my veins twice; that almost never happens. I then got an IV, and they missed that vein as well; that never happens. I was beginning to worry about the outcome. I do have to say, I was happy about the weight, but it looks like I shrunk an inch. Anyway, I'm going to leave that to their faulty equipment, because surely I could not have shrunk. Of course, I have to get completely undressed and they put on a gown that hooks up to a warmer, which was very nice. I remember to take off my underwear this time. Otherwise, they take it off for you and put it in a bag with a sticker with your name on it. It just reminds me that once on the operating table, everyone is the same piece of meat as the next guy, which is really a good thing. You don't want people getting all emotionally attached to you while they have your guts laying out on the table.

Next, the plastic surgeon enters. He has a little pouch of Sharpie pens to mark up where he's going to cut. I asked him if he got them at some special medical store—no, just Staples. I guess the latest and most advanced equipment wasn't used on me. I made sure that I told them I wanted even breasts. He said that he'd try. Also, my scar from when they took my expander out is stuck to my chest. I asked him if he was going to put his foot up on my chest to excise it from my chest wall. He laughed and said that he didn't think he'd have to do that. Next, the bartender came in to go over his speech. I asked him how long he has been doing this, and he said, "Since I was seven years old." So I told him that I will not be expecting to be missing any teeth by the time he gets done with me if he's been doing it that long.

Finally, I was wheeled into the operating room. The hallway was really cluttered with surgical supplies as was the actual operating room. Nothing like *Grey's Anatomy*. I guess at least everything is only an arm's length away. I didn't comment on that since the people in the room were about to cut me open. Next thing I know, I have the happy shot, and low and behold, I'm in the recovery room.

Once in the recovery room, I was really groggy from the happy morphine I got, but I swear that the nurse was hurrying me up to get me out of there. I did have the choice to stay overnight or go home. I wasn't feeling a lot of pain, so I opted to go home. Since it was a Friday afternoon, I don't think the nurse would have liked the paperwork needed for me to stay. I don't think I ever got dressed so quickly! They had me wheeled out of that joint quicker than I thought. However, I was half out of it, so time is kind of irrelevant when that happens. I don't really remember the ride home or much of the weekend to be honest. Dr. Plastic Surgeon only filled up my expander with 200cc compared with the 400cc from the last surgery. I'm obviously not in as much pain as last time. It's a little painful, but nothing like before.

I sent a fax to the doctor's office on Monday, letting Dr. Plastic Surgeon know that I was doing okay, except I was in a little bit of pain where he'd put his foot on my chest to get the scar off. I think he left a footprint. Actually, he cut out the scar and sent it to pathology. Everything came out fine. He even called me personally to see how I was doing. He said, "How is my young-looking patient?" Boy, I've got these doctors trained. I've been on pain pills and muscle relaxants for the past several days.

In the meantime, on Monday, I had a consultation with a new GYN about getting my ovaries out. This is the doctor that my breast surgeon had her hysterectomy from and my oncologist also knows. She was wonderful and much more laid back than the last one, and I didn't feel like I had to wear three-inch heels to visit the doctor. She asked when I wanted the surgery, and I asked what she was doing that afternoon. Apparently that's too soon to get things ready, but her surgery coordinator would be calling me. Like I said, I want all of this done by the end of the year. This doctor completely agreed with what my breast surgeon (who I assume is her buddy) said, so I had no argument from her about the surgery. It was actually a delightful experience, except for the scale. They didn't let me take half of my clothing off or shoes, so my weight that was higher than I would have liked.

Then this morning, my new best friend, the surgery scheduler, called and said that I was set for surgery on Monday, December 6th, at 11am. I have a pre-op appointment next Monday. I said, "Wow, you really are my new best friend for getting that on the schedule so fast." She replied that the doctor said I was a VIP and that we wanted it done as soon as possible. Dang. And I hardly did any training with this office on me being a favorite patient! How great is that?

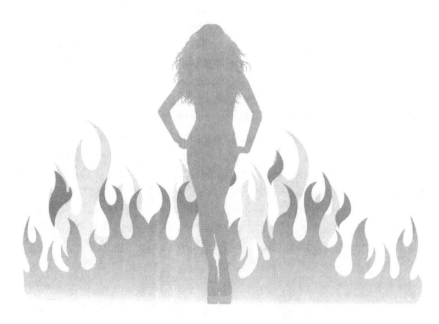

33 GIVING THANKS

November 25, 2010

This Thanksgiving is obviously a little more special than most of them I've had in the past for obvious reasons. I'm thankful for so many things. So much has happened this year that it's hard to know where to start to be thankful, but I'm going to try.

Dear Heavenly Father,

Thank you for giving me another year on this earth. It was looking a little bleak back in May, but thanks to You and the rest of the support team You sent me, I've made it through. Thank you for the reaction that my family had when they found out I was diagnosed with a rare breast cancer. My husband immediately said that we would take it out and get rid of it. He has stood by my side the whole time and never made me feel less than a woman or less of a person because of it. My parents had no problem flying across the country in a moment to be by my side.

Thank you for assembling the best team of doctors to help me fight the good fight of cancer. As soon as I walked into my breast cancer surgeon's office, I knew that she was the one. She immediately got on her cell phone and right there, after hours, scheduled appointments with her "team" for me for the next day. Thank you for the kindness and time that all of the doctors and their staff have taken with me. Some physicians took over two hours with me for the first visit. I have never felt like a number or "the cancer patient in room three." Thank you that You sent me people who are sincere and really truly seem to feel that they care about what happens about me. Whenever I've called my oncologist's office, I've always felt like they were responsive and had time to listen. Even the hospital staff have been wonderful, kind, and caring. Of course, I like to think that some of it has to do with my natural adorable nature, but I know that most of it's that You're watching over my care.

Thank you for the unexpected outpouring of love and caring from friends, co-workers, and family. This was quite unexpected. I can't tell You how often I would get an email from a friend "just checking in" and how much I really needed the boost that day. Thank You for those friends who would leave voicemail messages just to tell me they were thinking about me and not expecting anything in return—particularly because in the beginning, talking to anyone was way too emotional. I had no idea that I had that much love and support around me. I mean, I knew to some extent, but you never really know until something like this happens to you. Because of my cancer, I have made some friends that I know will be in my life for a very long time. I also have some friends who have always been in my life and just reassured me that they will continue to be part of my life for a long time. Sometimes, I sit back and can't believe how lucky I'm to have so many wonderful people in my life. Thank You for the people from my childhood who are supporting my parents. I have neighbors who helped to raise me who are praying for me. Thank You for all of the cards I've received from people who took the time out of their busy life to let me know that they were thinking about me, even though they hadn't seen me in years.

Thank You for my co-workers who immediately picked up my work and told me not to worry. Thank You for all of the love I have received from the workplaces that I have told. Thank You for all of the help I've received with the house, the kids, and when I've been ill. I've been truly blessed with our new home. It's like we moved into a place that embraced us without question. My husband has made friends. The kids' school has gone beyond the call of duty to help them out even without me having to be there every five minutes. They did it all because they cared.

Thank You for the patients I work with who I've told about my cancer and still want to wait to work with me. Although these patients are still patients, I believe that some of them have crossed the usual professional boundary and I can truly call them friends. I get texts asking how I'm doing from patients, friends, and family all the time.

I'm also blessed because in the midst of my life-battling struggle, this year, my cousin and sister-in-law are blessed with new babies. It reminds you how the circle of life comes full circle. Although having a disease like cancer makes you pretty selfish, I'm still thankful that they are experiencing the joy that comes along with having children.

I'm thankful, of course, for all of the material things that You continue to bless my family with. However, I have come to learn how little those things mean in the larger scheme of things. This year I've learned to trust and have faith that I do not have control over most things and that I have to let You take over. For someone who likes to be in control, have all of her ducks in a row and be organized, this has been a difficult lesson. But I have learned not to worry, things will work out. God will provide all that I need, whether it's finding the right treatment, doctor, getting the bills paid, or finding the right caretakers and therapists for my children. God will provide.

I'm thankful that I've learned the lesson that people have faults, scars, and are not perfect. Yes, that includes me. I knew that before, but I've really learned it this year. No matter what flaw a person has, that flaw does not mean that is all that they are. People are essentially the same inside when you take the time to look. Forgiveness is really not an option, but a way of living. Whatever gripes, disagreements, or arguments you have with someone, they're not worth holding on to. More importantly, it should not take a life-threatening illness to understand that. Sometimes we just need to agree that we disagree.

The other thing I'm thankful for is that I have learned to live in the moment. This moment is all we have. The energy I've wasted in the past worrying about what is going to happen or what is not going to happen could probably have fueled the space shuttle. I'm not saying that I have not shed plenty of tears over the past several months, but I have come to a place where I have learned that most things work out. The worst-case scenario usually doesn't happen. Another door usually opens—and it's usually a better one than we expected. I have learned that just when all hope seems lost, God sends us someone or some situation that gets us through. There are no coincidences. I have also learned that if the house is messy, the messy police do not show up. I have learned that if my kids' rooms are not perfectly organized, they're still able to function. I've even learned that living without hair does not make me less of anything. I'm still adorable—just minus the hair.

I've been blessed with a loving husband who, without hesitation, will hold me if I'm crying or sad, with wonderful children, and a supportive family. I live in a wonderful place and have friends who are there when I need them—even if it's just to listen to me vent. There is not much more than that.

Now that I'm cancer-free and am seeing the light at the end of the tunnel with my last operations, I'm even more thankful. Cancer has given me a chance to slow down and appreciate things that I hardly took notice of before. It's been difficult, but God has sent me all that I need to get through. I've faced the BIG C and conquered it. Yes, it might reoccur. Yes, it could come back and might come back even worse, or it might not come back at all. Either way, this is not for me to worry about. I truly believe, as I believe that every trial in my life has a purpose, that this cancer will one day reveal its purpose. Even if it doesn't, I've learned so much already. If God decided to take me up to heaven today, I'm ready. If he doesn't, then I know I have a lot more to do on this earth which has not all been revealed to me. I'm ready for whatever comes; I'm ready to take on whatever challenge that God sends me. I'm ready to be that rock for someone else. I'm ready to help others learn the same lessons that I have learned.

Thank you, Lord, for all that You've given me. Thank You for the very breath that I take each moment. Each one seems sweeter than the last these days. Thank You for all that you have given me. Thank You for my new mantra that God will provide. Through Jesus Christ. Amen.

By the way, I have also learned that having faith and sharing it with others is not politically incorrect and is sometimes just what someone else needs to hear.

Happy Thanksgiving.

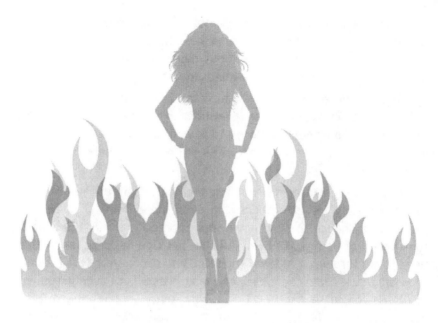

33 APPOINTMENTS WITH YOUR PARENTS

November 30, 2010

There's something about being 40 years old and having your parents come to your physician's appointments with you. I half expect my mother to pull out my little green book of immunizations to show the doctor. Since this is the breast doctor, my father waits in the waiting room. I love that he's concerned, but I'm still not going to have my dad watch while they fill my breast expander; there are limits. I've already had the big talk with my dad that I'm happy to take care of him when he's really old and needs help—but it will not be me wiping his butt. I will definitely be hiring some hot little nurse for him. I have my limits.

My rest on Sunday really started me back on my way to my old self. When we were in the waiting room at the plastic surgeon's office, it was me, my dad, and some other patient while my mom went to the restroom. When she came back from the restroom, I said loudly, "Boy, it doesn't look like you had a face lift. You might want your money back." The girls behind the desk snickered and my mother said the usual, "Real nice, Melissa."

Before going to the plastic surgeon's office, I stopped at Office Max to pick up a couple of things. It's the closest office supply store to my house and office, so I'm there fairly often picking up paper, toner, pens I don't need, you know, stuff like that. As soon as I walk in, someone always asks if I need any help. Usually roaming around paper products is nice enough for me, but this time I was looking for something specific. An older gentleman walked me over to the exciting pencil cases. He then went on to say that he hopes that he wasn't intruding, but he'd seen me in the store several times and he knows a woman who works with cancer patients. He was very genuine about it and handed me her card which had the title "Life Coach" on it. I despise that title, but that's a whole other conversation. I wanted to say, "Well, I'm a psychologist and have plenty of resources." Instead, I just said "thank you so much" and how thoughtful that was.

On one hand, it was very thoughtful and genuine. On the other hand, it confirmed that I'M the cancer lady when I go out to the few stores I frequent, which is basically Office Max, Target, the grocery store, and the McDonald's drive-thru. I figure as I start to feel better and before my hair grows in, I better start taking more advantage of the "cancer card" while I can.

Finally, we were called back, and my mom and I went back to the room. The woman who takes me back each time is really great and always takes time to talk with us. I never feel like I'm being rushed when I'm in the office. Of course, I'm sure it's because I'm their favorite and most adorable patient. This time around, Dr. Plastic Surgeon was MUCH more conservative. Last time he filled my expanders 400 ccs—this time I think he only did 100 ccs, so it's going to be a slow process getting me even again. The funny thing is, since my original breast surgery, I have no sensations in my breasts. I was getting something out of the oven the other day and realized that I was leaning on the oven door and didn't even feel it. Good thing I don't cook often. I was just heating up chicken nuggets.

Dr. Plastic Surgeon filled up my expander only 60ccs. So much for getting the implants done before the end of the year. Looks like we're taking things much slower than last time. This is probably a good thing, as it won't be as painful. I did ask for some more happy pills because it does still hurt; the muscle is being stretched. I pointed out that I sometimes get shooting pain in a particular place. The doctor explained that's probably where he'd had to put a suture. In addition, since I had a great big scar from when the original expander came out, the doctor really had to do some pulling and pushing. Ah, so that's the reason for the pain.

For the next several weeks, I will have to appear at the plastic surgeon's office so that they can continue to fill me up. My husband told me that I should ignore the office staff if they say that a mysterious person keeps calling and telling the doctor to fill me up so I have Double Ds. The fills do not hurt at all because again, I'm completely numb. Dr. Plastic Surgeon does not even use numbing medication. I don't even feel the needle going in; it's kind of a creepy thing for me to watch.

After this appointment, I was feeling pretty good because I got some more filling and my drain was removed. Those drains are really pretty painful and annoying. And for some reason, my daughter likes to try to grab it. When the doctor pulls it out, I'm surprised how long the tube is that's inside of me. Lovely. No wonder it's uncomfortable.

On to the gynecologist for my pre-operative appointment, with the parents in the car. How many of you can say that your father came with you to the gynecologist? I know you're jealous. Of course, he was remanded to the waiting room. I came in to the office with my Popcornopolis assortment in hand as a way of thanking them for getting me in so quickly and getting my surgery scheduled so soon. This particular doctor I really like. I like her mostly because my breast surgeon said she recently had a hysterectomy with her and who better to trust than another surgeon's opinion? The other reason is that it didn't appear that dressing like you just walked out of *Vogue* magazine was a requirement as a patient. Seeing that I have really only been wearing yoga pants since May, the fashionista hidden within me is not going to make an appearance anytime soon.

Within a surprisingly short period of time, I was called back—must have been the popcorn. I did let my mother come back with me since she was an OB/GYN nurse for most of her life. In case I forget to ask anything, she's there to back me up. Forgetting is a regular thing for me these days. As soon as we walk into the room, I let the nurse know that I need to use the restroom in case they need a urine sample. She tells me to go ahead and give one even though the doctor didn't ask for one yet. I just love these bathrooms with the instructions for the urine collections. To think that at least of page of instructions must be given to "pee in a cup" is really quite sad if you think about it.

My mom and I were really wondering why we were there. The doctor already saw me the week before. I just had a PET scan for her review and had surgery with the plastic surgeon the week before so she had all of that information. Well, guess what? This doctor actually wanted to take the time to go over the surgery time, procedure, risks and complications, post-surgery medications, and recovery times on her own. Wow. I don't think I even had anyone sit me down, let alone a doctor, and go over those things with my very first surgery in May. Again, Dr. Gyn was calm and took plenty of time with me. I never felt rushed at all. I also told her that once she got in there, if she saw anything strange to take care of it right then and there. Don't waste your time waking me up and discussing anything. I want all of this stuff done now. Apparently the plan is that I'm going to be in the hospital on Monday morning, surgery is at noon, and the plan is for me to stay at least one night. Recovery time varies, but she said to expect to recover at home for about one to two weeks. She did say that I could walk or use the treadmill as tolerated, so there goes my "no exercise" plan. From what I have heard from other cancer patients, this is probably the easiest surgery and procedure compared to the expanders and chemo itself. We'll see if that happens.

When the doctor was finished talking with me and going over all of the points of the surgery, her nurse walked in with a urine specimen container that was not the same color as what I had given earlier. Startled, I said, "are you actually bringing my pee back to me? If you don't need it, you can throw it out." She laughed at me and said that it was the special antibacterial soap that I needed to shower with the night before and the day of the surgery. Wow, free samples. I had to buy the stuff for my last surgery. I guess it's important to be extra clean for these things. My husband is excited because where I'm having surgery is RIGHT next to where he goes to Applebee's for poker every Monday night. I'm sure I'll have a room full of visitors the night after the surgery.

I realize I'm really trying to shove as much stuff in as possible before the end of the year. I'll probably have to be the director and not the doer for the Christmas decorating, as I'll be recovering from the surgery. My son is already ready to have the Christmas tree up. I'm just really trying to start 2011 out on the right foot. It seems like I've been living and breathing cancer for years now, even though it's only been since May. Once again, I'm going to have to pace myself with my recovery from this surgery. That part really sucks. It sucks not only because I feel weak and can't do much for very long, but it makes me think about getting old. This must be what it's like to get old; your mind wants you to do something, but your body isn't responding. Remind me that I actually do want to get really healthy and eat right after all of this is done.

Hopefully, my good spirits will last a while longer—at least until next Monday, when I have to go under the knife again to have a complete hysterectomy. The funny thing about getting breast cancer is you get used to having the word "breast" roll off your tongue without blinking an eye. I can even say it in front of my father without thinking about it. Breast this. Breast that. Breast. Breast. Breast. Now, hysterectomy and the parts involved in that are not rolling off my tongue as easily. I already know that several of my friends who are as "ancient" as I am are jealous I don't have the monthly visitor every month. That's excitement. Yes, I know. I will have to get out more once this is all done.

34 "IF I SHOULD DIE YOUNG..."

December 3, 2010

There's a new country song out called "If I Should Die Young". When I first heard it, I felt like I was rubbernecking at a car accident. I just couldn't turn it off. The song tells a story about a young girl describing how she wants things to go if she dies young. This is not a subject that I've openly explored. However, I'm pretty sure that every cancer patient and their family think about death as they go through this journey. As much as there is talk about "going for the cure" and "positive thinking" patients live longer, inevitably, I believe that the cancer patient and his or her family has the death issue in the back of their mind.

But really, we all do. I could go into the theories of existential psychology at this point, although it would excite me, I won't bore you. We are the only creatures on the planet that are aware of our own demise. Even people without a terminal or chronic illness think about death and what would happen. Unfortunately, that's the reason for many teenage suicides, but the teenager forgets they're not around to see what happens. Ultimately, life goes on. I learned that lesson early on—not related just to death, but to most situations.

Since I had the PET scan and was told that I'm cancer-free, I think I have a little more objectivity—well, as much as one can have in this situation about the reality of death. As the saying goes, "It's the ultimate equalizer. We all die eventually." This subject weighed heavy on my mind in the beginning, as I'm sure it did with those around me. Those first couple of months, I think that I was constantly asking myself, "Am I going to die? Is the cancer spreading? Will death be painful?" I don't think I said it out loud. I also know that my husband and family discussed it, but not in front of me, because I was going through the natural depression that occurs when someone tells you that you have cancer.

Even now, it's hard not to think that every ache or pain is not somehow related to cancer and if it has come back. How do you go back to living when you faced death so closely in the face? I think this is a hard question to deal with. I live now knowing, as my oncologist put it, that my body is capable of making cancerous cells. I can have a relapse. I can never have to deal with this again. It's really unknown. But I can't focus on that. I have way too much to do and way too much I plan to do.

I do have a strong faith and firmly believe that as another county song says, "It can't all end in a long ride in a hearse." I believe that I'm going to heaven and that if God takes me tomorrow, I, personally am okay with that. I read *90 Minutes in Heaven and* other books like it. I know that if this cancer was the way I was going to go, then I'm okay with it. It doesn't mean that I'm not going to fight it. I know there are lessons to be learned in every trial. I also know that in the future days, I will appreciate my family and friends more than ever and take time for more moments in my life instead of rushing.

That reminds me. I remember when I was younger, our church went from the "communal" communion cup to little plastic cups for the wine part of the sacrament in response to all of the AIDS and other health scares. I remember my mom saying that if God was going to take her because she got some disease taking communion from the communal cup, then so be it; He must really want her. I kind of take that same approach to things. If God really wants me because I got some terrible disease off the grocery cart, then you just know that it's your time to go. So far, I don't think God is taking me because of cancer... at least not this year.

One time I heard an interview with Dr. Wayne Dyer. For those of you who don't know who he is, he's an inspirational speaker with a degree in psychology. He has written many books and many of them have reflected is own personal journey. In this interview, he was asked how he'd like to remembered when he's dead. He paused for a moment and said, "I really don't care." I think that's probably one of the best responses I've heard. Once you're dead, you don't care. However, we all have a little narcissism in us and do hope that despite being one of billions of people on this earth, we'll have left a legacy, a mark, or an imprint that we were here. I can't necessarily say that I'm any different, but I do think that those of you who know me should have some guidelines in case the inevitable happens. Now, don't get me wrong. I fully plan on living to a ripe old age of at least 100. I plan on being an annoying old lady and probably dying while I'm working much to the horror of whatever therapy patient is sitting across from me. I plan on being a smart ass, sarcastic, and embarrassing old woman to my parents, husband, family, and children for as long as I can. I still have great things ahead of me. However, here are some do's and don't's just in case:

I don't care if you bury or cremate me; I'll be dead. The more economical and space saving way would be to cremate me. I'm sure that God can figure out how to put me back together, if necessary. If you do decide to cremate me, don't put me in an urn and put me on display in the house or under the bed. I'm pretty sure that my parents still have their cremated dog from over 12 years ago under their bed—I don't want to be next to the dog. I also don't want to be a conversation starter in the house. "And over here is my mom in this fancy vase." Also, there's no need to get some fancy ash holder. I'm not much of a "bling" person now, and certainly don't want a blinged-out urn. Instead, just get a box that hopefully the funeral home won't charge extra for, and spread my ashes somewhere. Any place peaceful, like the ocean, on top of a hill with a view, or a corn field in Illinois. Don't spread me some place where someone lives, then there will be the perpetual guilt that you can't sell the house because "Melissa's ashes are there." Go with someplace public.

Another option, of course inspired by a country song, would be to stuff me and prop me up by the jukebox and put a stiff drink in my hand. That one is kind of morbid and might be difficult to explain. But again, an option.

If you insist on burying me, I don't need a "special" location in the cemetery like a plot with a view or next to a bench. Again, I'll be dead and won't really care. I think this would be a tough one. My only concern is how to best deal with the whole death thing with my children—who, remember, have special needs. If you bury me and tell them I'm in the ground, they'll probably take it literally and then they'll freak out. I'd prefer that you tell them I went to heaven and am with them all the time. Also, if I'm buried, you don't need to come and visit. I'll be dead. I'm not my body. My soul will not be hanging out at the cemetery. I'll probably be haunting you part-time and then part-time in heaven.

A couple of other notes. If I die before all of my hair comes back in, there is no need to put a wig on me when I'm displayed. You can throw a hat on me like I have been wearing for the last couple of months. I feel like a drag queen in the wig that I have now. So I certainly don't want to look like one when I'm laid out. Also, you can bury me or cremate me in a white t-shirt. I have a closet full to choose from. Don't try to dress me up in some special outfit. Let's face it. My wardrobe now is white, black and tan. If you change it, no one will recognize me. Make sure all my jewelry is off. I have heard about people being buried with their jewels on. What a waste. I would rather have them sold on eBay than that.

Also, no one is to say, "She looks so good." If you think I look good when I'm dead and laid out in a casket, you better tell me now that I need a makeover; I won't be offended. But I can assure you, I'm not going to look better or good when I'm dead. If you have makeup suggestions now—please give them. You can put a note in my hand that says, "God, your favorite and most adorable child is on her way home to you." I would be okay with that.

If, for some reason, I do not die and am maimed or get brain damage from my upcoming surgeries, I have some more tips. Remember a couple of years ago, that woman in Florida was in a vegetative state and her husband and parents were fighting it out if they were going to keep her on life support or not? Well, if I have no brain function, it means the gray matter is NOT working. I'm not coming back to my usual perky self. I've taught physiological psychology. When the upper part of the brain is dead, so is the person. The brain stem just keeps you breathing. Don't put yourself through that. There are plenty of happy drugs that with the right overdose… well, you know what I mean.

However, as I mentioned when that whole Florida thing was going on—if for some reason, because of my adorableness, I end up on the news while in a vegetative state, for God's sake, put some makeup on me. I look like a hairless albino alien right now without makeup now and don't want to leave the house without some makeup. I certainly don't want to be on the evening news without it, either. Funny thing about that Florida story. The local news interviewed a mother whose beautiful daughter had brain damage and she was being cared for at home in a hospital bed. Guess what? That mother had the sense to throw some lipstick on her when the news crew came. That's what I'm talking about. I'm not completely vain but come on—a little blush never hurts.

My stuff. Again, I really don't care. I used to be really attached to my books, but now it doesn't matter. Things are just things and they can be replaced. I'll let my husband decide all of that; he'll know what to keep for himself and the kids. However, I will say that I have enough white t-shirts to go around that probably everyone could have one!

The obituary. I now live in a place where it seems like the obituary is like a literary piece of work. If you decide to do one—again, I don't really care, but here are some tips. Yes, use a picture of me with hair. Find the best one. Even for the obituaries that are from people who live to 100, I love seeing their young pictures. Feel free to take some artist embellishment license with it. If you write something like, "She loved scrapbooking and cats," or "She loved collecting spoons." I **will** come back to haunt you. I would rather it say something like "Melissa was adorable..." and so on. Again, feel free to really lay it out.

Finally, if you decide to have a memorial, funeral, whatever, then have some snacks. I hate going to funerals—especially the ones of relatives where I have to hang out most of the day—and not having snacks. Make sure they are good snacks. Remember, I'm the appetizer queen, so try to focus on that. I'm not talking about opening up a bag of tortilla chips and laying it on a table. Do what I do in these situations— call someone else to bring in the snacks. Get it catered—you can spend money on that. Good food is always worth it. I don't expect you to do extra work. And for God's sake, have some alcohol there. I'm a good German-Irish girl and would rather have the traditional Irish wake. No one likes going to funerals or wakes, so the alcohol will liven it up. I always think about the time that I drove my brother and his friends down to Chicago on St. Pat's day to go out. On the way down there, no one said a word. Once the first drink came, all of a sudden I couldn't get anybody to shut up. Alcohol definitely has its advantages in certain situations. And of course, country music needs to be playing.

If you feel the need to have a plaque or something to commemorate my life, I think the perfect solution would be a brick at Disneyland. It's the happiest place on earth. My kids love it and it has special memories for my husband. Feel free to put "Melissa the adorable one" on it or something like that. I'm good with that.

I will be dead. Do what you want. Do what is going to help you through it. As I said, I think some conversations need to happen. I've already talked with my parents that if they become incapacitated and need to have their asses wiped, as much as I love them, I will be hiring someone. I told my dad I'll find him some little hottie to take care of him. You see, if you discuss these things ahead of time, there's no fighting or arguing. When my parents get out of line, I remind them that there are the good nursing homes and then there are the bad ones— which one do they really want to go to? Also, I already told my husband if he goes senile, I'll be there for him, but each time I put in the same movie for him, I'll exclaim, "Look at the new movie I got you."

In all seriousness, if something does happen to me, I would ask that all of you form that village to help my children. My children have special needs and will have a harder road than most kids, even with an adorable mother by their side. Please tell my children fond memories you have of me (make some up if you have to), so that my memory is always with them. Remind them that even if I'm gone, I'm with them. Take time to spend time with them even if just for a couple of minutes. Send them birthday cards and sign that you were a friend of their mother's. However, I will say again that I do not plan on leaving this earth anytime soon. Even before the cancer, I believed and continue to believe that God placed those two precious souls in my care for a reason. I doubt he is going to take me until the job is done.

Oh, and one last thing. If I do die young (amazing what one country song can do for me), and you can't find your keys and then suddenly find them, find a great parking spot, the lights flicker, or things mysteriously move—it was probably me.

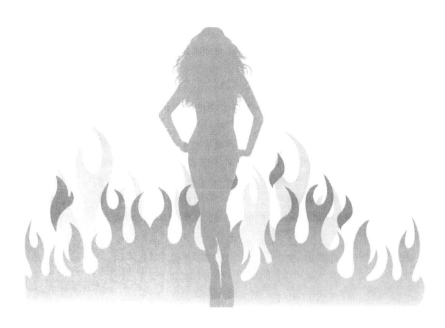

35 HYSTERECTOMY

December 11, 2010

On Monday, I had a complete hysterectomy laparoscopically. I had to stay in the hospital overnight. With all that I've been through over the past several months with the pain, drugs, fatigue of chemotherapy, and the all-over general feeling of malaise, I have been walking around telling everyone, "These last surgeries are going to be the least of it." Well. That is partly true, but not completely.

Prior to my surgery I had a pre-operative appointment with my surgeon. She even had a handout to go over what to expect about the surgery, which I thought was pretty cool because a lot of surgeons don't have a handy dandy one-page handout to give out. She went over how I was going to be in the hospital for at least 24 hours and the recovery would be about one to two weeks at home. She went over the usual things to call for like a high fever, excessive bleeding, etc. I was not to pick up anything heavier than a gallon of milk. During her talk, I kind of treated it like you do after you have been flying for a while. When the plane starts to take off and the flight attendants go over the safety features, the exits, and the life vests, you tune them out because you've heard it so many times. That's kind of how I felt. I've been poked, prodded, scanned, X-rayed, and pretty much been a human scientific project for the last several months. What's one more surgery?

Remember, I also do weight loss surgery evaluations, which are done laparoscopically. So, when I talk to patients about how the lapband is placed on the stomach, recovery time is almost nothing.

Monday morning as I was packing to go to the hospital, I brought a number of things to entertain myself such as my computer, books, and iPad. I wanted to be prepared so that heaven forbid I should be bored. I was actually impressed by the surgery center's efficiency. As soon as I checked in, I was whisked to the registration desk. After check-in, I hardly had a chance to sit down before the nurse called me back to get ready for surgery.

Funny thing. Lately there have been several billboards around town that have this particular hospital system advertising how "They take your cancer personally." Alongside that, there's a nurse that actually works at the hospital on a name badge that says, "Breast Cancer Survivor." I've really noticed these billboards for the obvious reason, but also because I used to be involved in some marketing for a surgery center and thought it was a clever idea. Well, sure enough, "Kelly" from the billboards was my pre-operative nurse. I thought I recognized her, but then one of her colleagues joked with her as we walked back that she saw her billboard again. I was quite excited because she had her hair back in a ponytail! Her hair had grown back! I said to her, "Wow your hair looks like it really came back great. How long did it take?" She then proceeded to tell me that she never had chemotherapy but she did have a mastectomy, reconstruction, and hysterectomy so her hair never fell out. Bummer, and I was so excited. She did have a very nice bejeweled pink ribbon name badge holder that was kind of cool.

She led me to a room where she instructed me to take off all of my clothes and put on the gown and socks. The hospitals now have these cool gowns that hook up to a vacuum-like machine and keep you warm. This part of the drill I knew well because if you recall, I left my underwear on during my first surgery. They came back to me in a baggie labeled by a sticker with my name on it. Apparently, once you're in the operating room you're just a body. And, it's hard to wear underwear when you have a catheter.

After getting naked and putting on my heatable gown, I was led to a bed where I was asked all the regular questions, had my blood drawn, and had the IV inserted. Standard stuff for me at this point. I was excited that the IV was going to be in my arm and not my port that was recently removed. The things I find exciting lately really scare me. I was telling my celebrity billboard nurse how both nurses in my last surgery had ended up sticking me twice and really had to dig for my veins, which generally doesn't happen. She explained to me that after chemotherapy, your veins can be more fickle and not as resilient as they once were. Just when I think that my use of denial as a defense mechanism is really working, I'm reminded that chemotherapy actually takes a toll on the body. Not that I don't get that reminder often because of my lingering body aches and lack of stamina—oh, and not having any hair is also a denial killer.

Next, the usual parade of doctors come in to visit me. First, the anesthesiologist. He looked like he was 20 years old. I joked with him that I hoped this wasn't his first time doing this. He laughed nervously, so I wasn't quite convinced, but I was happy to see that he already had the happy shot with him. He was just waiting for me to sign all of the consents and meet with the surgeon. Finally, the surgeon entered. She came in with her shoes covered in surgical booties and her keys in the other hand. It kind of made me feel like I was just a stop on her list of errands for the day. She didn't have a briefcase. Just her keys. That's someone who has it together—or maybe she forgot everything in the car. I went with the theory that she knew what she was doing. She explained the procedure to me again. And again, I kind of tuned it out. I was making my usual sarcastic jokes as we went along.

The nursing staff started to wheel me into the operating room. More importantly, the Bartender, as he is known to staff, or the anesthesiologist, gave me the happy shot. Once in the operating room, the nursing staff had the music blaring. There is so much stuff in the operating room, and I don't mean equipment, I mean stuff. Most of the shelves have gauze and instruments. I wonder how they get around in there. Finally, I'm asked to scoot onto the thin operating table and they start to strap me down. I slowly transfer from a chatting, adorable person to a piece of human flesh that's about to be cut. After that, I don't remember anything at all.

The next thing I know, I'm in the recovery area. To be honest, I hardly remember it. I was really in and out of it. I don't remember the nurse. I remember my husband coming in and telling me that the doctor told him that everything went well and that I'm okay. That is it.

This particular surgery center is a free standing center with nine beds on the second floor. That is where I would be staying for the night. The celebrity billboard nurse said there were plasma screen televisions and made it sound like I was going to be in a spa. Well, I think they forgot the plasma screen television in my room. It wasn't even a flat-screen. The room was very nice, but I have to tell you, my memory of the whole first day after the surgery was very blurry. Of course, I was cognizant enough to tell the nurses to keep the drugs coming. At this point, one wonders why I packed anything at all to come to the hospital. I was completely out of it and had a catheter, so I wasn't going to be roaming the halls looking for the gift shops.

Much to my dismay, with the catheter in, my nurse came in soon after surgery and made me do laps around the unit—and not to look for the gift shops. She did this several times, even in the middle of the night. That was fun. No makeup, a gown that opened in the back, an IV pole and a catheter—far from the beauty pageant walk. Thank God she was with me when we did the walk, because I was really pretty unsteady. I didn't sleep that much while in the hospital because of the noise, the walking, and my vitals being taken every two minutes. I do have to say that the food was good. I was given a three-ring binder and told that I could order whatever I wanted, whenever I wanted. Of course, this would have been great if I'd been hungry.

In the morning, my surgeon came in to tell me everything went fine and that I could be discharged. If I wasn't able to urinate on my own, she would send me home with a catheter. Yeah, that wasn't going to happen. I ordered a latte and started to power drink so that I'd pee. Again, see how the excitement in your life can change when you have a major illness. Why I packed all that crap to keep myself occupied, I'll never know. I don't think that I even opened my backpack except to get dressed to get home. I never even turned on the television. I did eventually pee on my own. I was really still hopped on all of the IV drugs, so when my husband picked me up to leave, I was feeling pretty good. If you can believe it, we actually went to Applebee's for lunch before heading home. We were definitely the youngest people in the entire place. I thought it was senior special day but, no, it was just an average Tuesday afternoon. I did have to ask my husband several times what day it was.

Once I got home, I was still feeling pretty good. I had my Vicodin and went to bed. The rest of the night was a complete blur. Thank goodness for my husband and my babysitter. So, soon after I got home, I started to learn that just because a surgery is laparoscopic doesn't mean NO recovery time. Soon, it became apparent that, yes, indeed, I did have a major surgery, although it was hard to tell because I only have three little openings on my belly, I mean my six-pack of abs. That was the other thing, I kind of expected to have a fabulously flat stomach after the surgery. After all, when you take parts out, you'd think that things would flatten out a bit. But, again, they do blow up your abdomen with air so they can see the surgical field. As a result, my stomach is even more extended than usual. As the pain pills started to wear off, it felt like someone had kicked me in the stomach.

On Wednesday, I started to get a low-grade fever. I left a message for the doctor and, believe it or not, she called me back herself. She explained to me that my fever was not much of a concern unless it got really high. It was due to the inflammation related to the surgery. She reminded me that I'd just had a complete hysterectomy, which is pretty major surgery, and I should probably be resting—like she told me before the surgery—that must have been when I was spacing out like I do on plane rides.

■

For most of the week, I've been up in the morning. Well, getting out of bed while moving extremely slowly, taking a pain pill, and then trying to get some work done. The rest of the day is spent lying down, wondering why I'm not running a marathon yet —after all, wasn't this supposed to be the easy part of the treatment? I think I was still constantly asking my husband what day it was.

On Thursday, I did have an appointment with the plastic surgeon to get more saline in my expander. I didn't have a pain pill that morning so I could drive myself. It felt like a milestone, but I suffered for it later. The appointment was at 9:30am, so I was not a happy camper. I usually try to bring the staff snacks since I'm the favorite patient, but I was pretty lucky just to be there.

Once again, Dr. Plastic Surgeon started to fill my right expander. My breasts are so numb that he didn't even need a numbing agent as he put the large needle in my breast. I didn't even really feel it. He then used what was probably a horse syringe from the veterinarian down the street to add fluid. I finally felt some pressure from the fluid and he stopped. I'm actually starting to look even. I still have about two fills to go before I can have the implants switched out. Unfortunately, my plan to have all of my surgeries done by the end of the year probably won't happen because of the holidays. I will have to wait for the first or second week of January, so 2011 will be the year of the new perky breasts. Apparently, THAT surgery is supposed to be no big deal and is done on an outpatient basis, where you go home the same day. I'll believe that when I see it.

This one appointment completely wore me out, so I went directly back home to take more pain pills and go to bed. Now, not only did I feel like someone had kicked me in the stomach, my chest felt completely tight as my muscles started to spasm from the fill. Sounds like fun. I know you're jealous.

My gynecologist called herself to check on me. Again, I get a little freaked out. When the doctor calls and not one of her assistants, there has to be something urgent. She told me that my pathology reports came back completely normal, so I have nothing to worry about regarding cancer in my reproductive system. She asked how I was doing, and I told her that I was still in pain, tired, and wouldn't be running any marathons soon. She again reminded me that I'd just had major surgery. In the "old days", women would stay in the hospital for a week after a hysterectomy and then would be on six weeks' bed rest at home afterward.

I finally started to get the idea that my recovery from surgery would be a very long journey. Not to mention, my body is still recovering from the chemotherapy. This is evident because I have lost more eyelashes and eyebrows in the last couple of weeks. This completely sucks because I'm so bad at drawing on eyebrows. I feel like Tammy Faye Baker when I do. I stopped using the expensive shampoo that I bought that's supposed to help with hair growth and thickness for "even chemotherapy patients." No sense using it if I'm still losing hair.

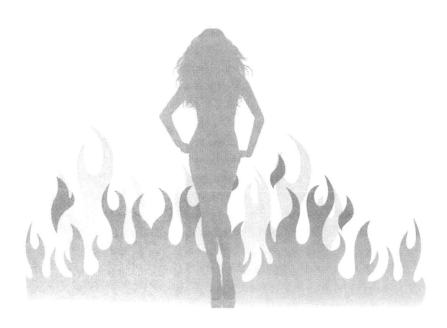

36 BALD ALBINO

December 13, 2010

My chemotherapy has been over since October 20th. The hope has been that my hair would start growing back. This morning I wake up and look like the albino Uncle Fester from the Adams Family. I have almost no eyebrows! What the F*&%!!!!

I thought the hair loss thing was over. But my eyelashes are barely hanging on! That is really upsetting because whenever I'm asked if I was stranded on a remote island, what is the one thing I would bring, I always answer mascara! Well, if I have no eyelashes to put the stuff on, what good is mascara? It wouldn't be that bad if I was better at putting on eyebrows. Since I'm so fair, I've never really had to "shape" my eyebrows or do a whole lot with them. I tried drawing them on this morning and I looked wide awake. I had to start over. Of course, as I was on bed rest over the weekend, one of the things a magazine said is to make sure that you accentuate your eyebrows as you get older. If you don't, you look even older. I had to run an errand yesterday and you can bet that my hat was lower than usual.

I'm starting to feel better, slowly but surely, but the appearance is not improving. Well, I can't completely say that. As my expanders are filled up, I look more even in the chest area. This is good, except that with the right expander, which is still getting its fills, I'm getting "side boobies." Until I'm completely filled, the breast won't be perky. I made it perfectly clear to Dr. Plastic Surgeon that I DO NOT WANT side boobies.

For those of you who do not know what that is, it's when your breast tissue wanders off to the side toward your underarm. This make for a difficult time finding a bra, not to mention a swimsuit. Maybe I should have a shirt made that says "No Side Boobies" for my next fill which is on Thursday. However, I do think that I have already made my point with Dr. Plastic Surgeon. Here is a tip: If you ever get breast augmentation, reduction, or reconstruction, it's always best to be nice to the surgeon. After all, if he doesn't like you, when you're on the operating table, you're helpless. So, I always bring snacks to my visits.

This week, Elizabeth Edwards died of breast cancer. Wherever you first get "the cancer", that's what it's called—in her case breast cancer, even if it comes back somewhere else like the liver. That is the scary part—cancer can metastasize years later. From what I read, she died the day after she stopped having treatments because they figured there was nothing else to do about it. Now, I remember thinking about what an ass her husband, John Edwards, was for cheating on her "while she was in remission", and then he had a love child with the woman. The stories definitely bring a feeling of loneliness that breast cancer causes its victim.

I'm on an email list for psychologists in the area. The latest message over the weekend was how one of the "beloved psychologists" in the state died of breast cancer. She was diagnosed five years ago and it metastasized to her bones, lungs, and liver. As you probably know, with a list serve, people can press "reply to all" and give their comments. So all weekend, whenever I turned on my computer, I got to hear about this wonderful woman and her fight over the past five years. As someone who just got the okay that I'm cancer-free, these stories really are a mere reminder of the strength of cancer.

On one hand, I hear stories of women who had breast cancer once and it never came back and they live to be annoying old ladies. Then there are these stories: Only five years ago, she got her initial diagnosis and now is dead. Now, the academic in me tries to remember that every case is different. Early detection saves lives. I don't know how far along these women were when they first got treatment or if they went through with all of the treatment that was recommended. The emotional side of me says "Holy S*$T!"

I mean, what if I've gone through all of this—surgery and chemo—and it comes back? Of course, I don't want to think about it and want to be positive, but it's a reality. I'm reminded that the doctors are going to be following me for the rest of my life, and there will be more scans and blood tests, but is that enough?! Why hasn't someone invented something like what radiologists wear to indicate if they are being exposed to too much radiation from their job? I would go for a "cancer gauge implant." The implant would alert you if your body started making cancer cells again. It would be like an alarm that would go off. This would help with the in-between visits to the doctors. How do you really know? Not to mention that I have a "weird" cancer that is only one percent of all breast cancers. I guess I should say "had cancer" because apparently it's gone. Is cancer ever really gone after it has made its mark?

Why did this happen to me? What is the future going to look like? What about my daughter, is she going to get it? Was this just a one-time thing that I have to deal with because I prayed for patience? Be careful what you pray for; you just might get it. If I did get it again, would I have the physical and emotional strength to go through chemo again?

I have chemo fog for many things, but when I hear that someone has died because of breast cancer, all of a sudden my mind perks up. Of course I'm going to use my psychological powers for good on myself. I'll remind myself that I can't worry about the future. The doctors said they got all the cancer. I have done everything humanly possible to prevent a re-occurrence.

I don't know how other cancer "survivors" deal with this kind of stuff but I do imagine that "cancer" is always in the back of their mind. I have read stories that the first mammogram after being in treatment can be the most emotional. Not only that, but I wasn't someone who was chronically sick—if you don't count college and when I was trying to get into graduate school—that was mostly psychosomatic illnesses, so they don't really count. Other than having my kids, Robitussin solved most of my problems. Now I'm going to forever be a patient. I'm labeled for life.

This will really give me sympathy for my own therapy patients and actually fits right in with my health psychology training. On the other hand, it just sucks. As I have found out this year, having medical issues is a full-time job. Even as I plan out the New Year, I have to consider when I have to fit in to see my doctors. That reminds me—I have to fit in my kids' doctor and dentist appointments also! So much to do.

Finally, as the holidays approach, I've been getting Christmas cards in the mail like I do every year. I'm going to work on them myself. I haven't been good at them in the past. I'm usually so busy that sending cards seems like a chore. Besides, we have the internet. A couple of clicks and I can send an e-card to everyone. But let's face it, everyone likes getting a real piece of mail. Also, if you recall, I asked my breast surgeon if she was still getting Christmas cards from her patients who had metaplastic cancer. She said she was getting several. Now sending out holiday cards almost seems like a way to let people know that I'm still alive! I guess I better go get some stamps.

I've been trying the whole vitamin and protein shake thing, and it doesn't seem to help! What's up with that? I guess all of this just takes some time. So, I've been in bed for a good portion of the last five days. Good thing I like my sheets.

37 NO DISNEYLAND

December 17, 2010

Yesterday, I had my appointment with my plastic surgeon where he filled up my expander again. Now I have almost two huge rocks on my chest. Sleeping on my stomach is not an option. At least I'm looking more symmetrical. But dang, they are sore. Apparently he had to stitch in a "hammock" of sorts and those sutures are causing me some pain. Just imagine walking around with two boulders on your chest and you'll get the idea. And to top that off, those boulders have to stretch your muscles in the meantime. Feels real good. My husband offered to massage them for me if I wanted—because he's nice like that—but I can barely touch them. He actually asked me if they still had about a gallon of fluid to put in each breast. He was just kidding—at least, I hope.

I have one more fill of the right expander next week. And then, guess what? He could switch out the expanders for the implants as early as two weeks. BUT since I was without an expander for so long he feels it's best to wait to have the surgery until LATE JANUARY! I've been bringing the surgeon and his staff gifts every visit—you'd think they could magically get things done for me. Medicine—sometimes I just gotta wonder, is it really a science? But seriously, I guess it's better to wait.

I'm just disappointed because once again, I thought in my head I would be back to Perky Missy (not just in the chest, by the way, but just in general) by the end of December. It's not going to happen.

Since I've been feeling so exhausted and am tired and achy all over, I called my oncologist's office to basically yell at them as to why I'm not better yet. I was hoping for some magic answer to solve all of my problems, like eat seven servings of broccoli or something. The medical assistant said that all of that was normal. I ended up playing phone tag with the physician's assistant. Probably a good thing I didn't get him; I either would have bitched him out or started crying, which I really hate doing. I waited until I got home to cry to my husband, who told me just to take it easy and lay down, so I did.

I mean, even my forearms ache. What's up with that? It really sucks. I feel like an old lady. Getting up in the morning takes a while. I really need my coffee to get going. And then, of course, there are the hot flashes. They've gotten worse. Nothing better than having your head start to literally sweat when you're out in public. I'm really trying to stay positive here, but it's been tough this past week.

Today didn't start out much better. Kids and cancer don't seem to mix either. I guess I should start to say "recovery from cancer" since my PET scan was clear. It's all about how you think, right?

My daughter woke up at 6am and wanted to watch *Playhouse Disney*. I tried getting her back to sleep so I could get one more precious hour of sleep myself. She was having none of it. Oh well, I had to get up and get cute to go to my 8:45 doctor's appointment with the GYN who did my hysterectomy. I'm sure that must have been the last appointment they had, because I really try not to have to face doctors these days before 10am.

I got my daughter set up doing puzzles, eating breakfast, and watching television. Well, as I'm taking a shower, she decides to go to my desk and pour out almost a whole bottle of nail polish on my desk. Thank goodness it wasn't on my computer keyboard. She has to be watched every minute! As soon as I turn my back, she has my chair pulled over to the cupboards to get more stuff. She is a quick one. In the meantime, my son is yelling, "She's from another planet! It's not morning yet! Make her go to bed!"

It was such a relaxing morning. And to think, today is their last day of school for two weeks.

Once I get to the doctor's office, of course, everyone is so nice. Unfortunately, I really had to put on my adorable act, since I was feeling like crap. The nurse calls me back and puts me on the damn scale. Is it really necessary to weigh me every time? I was going to be one of those women who takes off their shoes and jewelry and everything, but I left my shoes on and decided "What the hell does it matter?" I have those big Sketchers Shape-ups, so I usually account for at least five pounds for that. Once in the room, my GYN has gone hi-tech. There's a Mac monitor with information from everything from birth control to self-breast cancer exams. I have to say it way pretty cool, except that none of the topics applied to me. There was no topic, "Just had a hysterectomy to prevent future cancer?" but it was pretty cool and a great distraction while I waited for the doctor.

After we began talking, I started to tear up a little bit, saying that I'm not used to feeling this run-down all the time. Instead of giving me the magic pill or waving a magic princess wand over me, she told me the same thing: I need to rest. I should be on bed rest for at least another week, just to get back to baseline chemo achiness and fatigue level. I asked her every way possible to see if she would give me a different answer. She just shook her head and said that I would get back to feeling normal eventually, but not right now. Right now, I need to rest.

I then mentioned that my husband and I were thinking about taking the kids to Disneyland between Christmas and New Year's Eve. I told her that even I thought that would be a lot for me. She looked at me like I was crazy and said, "I usually don't tell people flat out NO, but NO Disneyland or anything like it for a while."

Can you believe I was told NO Disneyland?! She must really mean that I have to rest. She reminded me that if I do not rest I'm more susceptible to illness, and then I would be even worse because my immune system will be compromised.

What about if I just start drinking Gatorade or whatever those athletes take to give them more endurance? Maybe that would work. I started taking a bunch of supplements, but I still prefer chocolate when my stomach can handle it. The problem with the athletes supplements is that if I'm not working out, I probably would gain a bunch of weight. Then I would be really depressed.

Finally, good news on the hair growth front. Although my eyebrows and eyelashes seem to be leaving me, my hair is starting to bud back. I have hair follicles with actual tiny pieces of hair coming out of my head! I guess I'll start using the shampoo I bought.

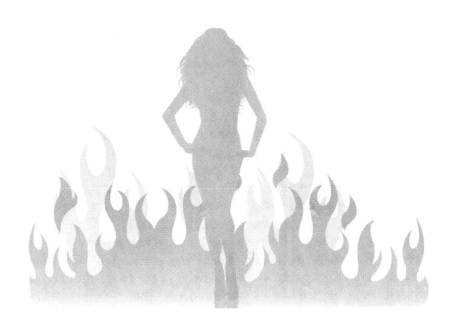

38 NO VOICE

December 20-22, 2010

You're not going to believe this, but I've lost my voice this evening. When it rains, it pours. I mean, at least the adorable cancer patient can talk. I'm using all the remedies in the book so at least I have my voice back. I'm sure it's not related to anything even remotely close to what I've been going through, but nonetheless annoying. I was actually feeling pretty good today, and then my voice goes out. I was talking too much! Imagine that. I have *never* been accused of that.

My husband had a Christmas party for his poker friends. I wasn't supposed to do anything except make chili. Well, we all know how that goes. I ended up doing more than I was supposed to, and then I started to play poker! I actually came in fourth place! I thought that was pretty good. I tried to bluff by taking off my hat and saying that they were taking money away from my chemotherapy treatments. It was actually a lot of fun. Maybe I can become the next Annie Duke, World Series of Poker champion.

That being said, I stayed up later than I have since probably January. I did more than I was supposed to, and I suffered dearly for it. I was in bed all weekend. On Sunday, I was so achy and exhausted, I was in tears. It was horrible. Ah, but the magic of drugs. Today I got my pain pills refilled and took it easy.

You'd think that by this time I would learn, but no. It takes me a while.

■

I finally went to the doctor after Nurse Hatchet told me to go. I've had so much tea and lemon, I think I'm drowning in it. I can now understand the secret reason behind the real tea party, where they dumped it all into the sea. Too much tea is not a good thing. As you can imagine, there are several people in my household who think the idea of me not being able to speak is to their liking. I tried to answer my phone a couple of times and people were like, "WHO IS THIS?"

I decided to go to the doctor to see if I could take a pill to make this go away. Annoyingly, my regular doctor was not available, so I saw a perky physician's assistant. She was actually really good, but I'm sure I was older than her, thus this was annoying. Then with my obvious appearance, she had to go into how her mother had breast cancer, so that took about 30 minutes. She gave me some antibiotics, but basically said it was viral and my ears looked a little full. She only gave me the antibiotics because my whole body has been a science experiment for the last year. But then, guess what she recommended? REST and not talking. What the hell is the resting thing?!

Actually, I find this to be a sign from God because if I can't talk, I can't work. Silence perhaps can be an absolute blessing. After all, talking is a big part of what I do. This must be a sign that I need to slow down. I do have to admit that other than my voice being gone, I feel pretty good. This is probably, and I hate to admit this, because I've spent the last five or more days resting. Go figure; maybe it does work, but it's still annoying. It's annoying also because I still don't have any concentration, so it's not like I'm reading some fabulous non-fiction book. And, to be honest, even reading gossip magazines, I don't know who the hell the people are anymore as I don't watch a lot of television and I especially don't watch reality shows. Except *Pawn Stars*; I like that one.

Although I wasn't able to talk, I did run a couple of errands today. I wanted to get some stocking stuffers for the kids—like they don't have enough to play with already. However, I've learned my lesson; it's just the opening that's fun. My son still has toys on his shelf not opened from last year. I went a little overboard last year, so here I am in the wrapping aisle in Walmart and a woman passes by the aisle and makes a point to come up to me.

She introduces herself and tells me that she was approached once when she was bald from cancer treatments. She was really sweet. She also had a nice head of hair and let me know that it does grow back, and things do go back to normal. She had me crying—well, tearing up—for the record, I didn't go into a full-blown crying jag—in the middle of Walmart. I know that there really is this sisterhood of women who've had breast cancer, but I guess I'm just not at that point yet where I want to admit it. I'm really enjoying my denial as a defense mechanism. I know that's going to eventually change. I know that this is happening to me for a reason. I know that one day it'll be revealed to me, but I guess I'm just not mentally ready for that since I'm still in the midst of it.

I wanted to get a friend of mine some manicure items as a Christmas gift along with the stuff that disinfects the tools. Long story. Anyway, I walk into Sally Beauty Supply, and you should have seen the look that I got from the girl behind the counter. It was the smiling face that was sweet, but probably thinking, *What the heck are you doing here?* After I got all the supplies, I asked her about fake eyelashes. I plan on eventually getting dressed up at some point, so I figure I'll need some. She picked out a starter kit for me. Did you know that you generally do NOT put them on the bottom lid? The things I don't know about beauty products amaze me.

Good news on the hair growth front! I'm getting significant fuzz on top of the head and I even saw some sprouts on my legs. I could do without shaving my legs, but the hair on my head is good. My eyebrows even look like they are coming back, but it's such baby fine hair that it doesn't really pass for eyebrows. I have been trying to pencil in the eyebrows, but I don't seem to be improving with practice. Oh well. At least some progress is being made.

Tomorrow, I go to my plastic surgeon to get my last fill in my expander before surgery. I cannot wait to have the implants. These expanders are killing me. No presents for them tomorrow! I hope to schedule a possible surgery date as well.

Finally, I think I've mentioned that I get hot flashes. Well, since my ovaries have been removed—they've been HORRIBLE. I woke up the other night with my shirt literally drenched. That was pleasant. I don't think I've slept a full night since this all started because as soon as chemotherapy started, I went into fake menopause. I went and stocked up on evening primrose oil. I will probably be doubling the dose. Not having a period is great, but dang, I never know if I'm hot or cold. I dress in layers. And my head starts to sweat, which is okay when you're bald, but I can just imagine how this is going to work once I have hair again.

39 A HOPEFUL & HAPPY
NEW YEAR

December 27, 2010 — January 3, 2011

Today, I'm recovering from chasing my two children around for two solid days. On Christmas Eve, we went to a friend's house for appetizers and drinks! Yes, I did have a glass of wine and damn, did it hit me hard. I'm going to have to build up the old German-Irish tolerance I once had. The kids had a great time opening their gifts. I didn't go overboard this year like I have in the past. Partly because of less cash-ola, but more because they have so much stuff already!

My voice finally came back, much to the dismay of my family.

I'm wondering if one can overdose on evening primrose oil. These hot flashes, especially at night, are killing me. I certainly hope this is not going to go on forever. It's like I can't get my body temperature or the room temperature regulated.

My hair is starting to fuzz up. This is the good news. Now, the bad news All of my eyelashes have fallen out. I have my fake ones, which you're only supposed to wear about five times. Thus, this makes me have to make the decision about what is a "lash-wearing worthy" event. Certainly not a trip to the grocery store or Target, but to be honest, I've never even tried wearing fake ones. I'll probably have to look up on YouTube how to apply these things.

Everything seems to be going well. I got my last fill in my right expander last week. So, of course, it's now killing me! My surgery to have the implants put in is on January 21, 2011. Apparently that surgery is supposed to be pretty easy. They do the nipples several weeks later and then tattoo them several weeks after that. I don't even want to know how they do it, but of course, they are both in office procedures, so I'll have a good view of it. I wonder if the doctor even uses topical anesthesia. That area of my chest is so numb when he fills them, he doesn't use anything at all. I don't feel anything.

Here's more information that you don't want to know, but it comes with the package. I've started bleeding from the hysterectomy. I called my doctor and have to go in and see her tomorrow. It's not an emergency, but I'm going to be really pissed if I have to have another surgery because of a complication or something. I'm trying to think positive and it's probably nothing. Of course, this delays my plan to start exercising every day because I have to be resting until I see her. That's really too bad, now isn't it?

I've been spending quite a bit of time rubbing my fuzzy head. My hair is growing back in and think I see a natural color of reddish blond coming up. My eyebrows also. It's quite exciting. However, I do feel like I'm looking a little strange with the hair coming back. I feel like I need the wig more now. It looks like I'm in-between wanting a bald head or a little like how Demi Moore looked like in *GI Jane*—of course, if I had the body to go with the look, I would be fabulously happy.

The problem with being on bed rest is the boredom. Usually when I'm really bored, I eat. I don't want to do that. I lost a couple of pounds and don't want to put them back on—but we still have a lot of candy from Christmas. So hard to avoid! I wasn't able to eat chocolate during chemotherapy, but my love affair with each morsel is getting so dangerously good. My stomach has not completely recovered—I can't do spicy food at all. I also haven't had Diet Coke in months other than once in a great while, or if I've gone out to a restaurant. I used to have a supply on hand all the time. I drink mostly water. Who would have thought that I would cut back on Diet Coke like that? I mean, I used to have a 32 ounce cup of it next to me at all times.

■

Goodbye 2010 and Hello 2011. I'm hoping for a much better year this year. This season of my life is hopefully coming to a close in the next several months. I was hoping that it would be over by today, but it looks like I still have to get my hair back and have a couple more surgeries. I still have to rest. I don't have the stamina or the energy that I thought I would by this time.

If I didn't get care at an early stage, then I would have been much worse off by this time. I've been at this for eight months now. I'm thankful for so many things despite my bad days and complaining. I have been truly blessed.

Eight months have gone by, just like that, like being pregnant and waiting for that new life to bless us. This was the birth of a new me. It's hard to believe that this all started with a phone call from my doctor on May 4, 2010 in front of the mailbox place. It's amazing how one phone call can change your life. Of course, it would nice if the lottery called and changed my life, but I guess I got a different kind of phone call. This year has been quite a challenge in many ways. I feel like I have missed almost a year of my kids' lives. Thankfully, we have a wonderful babysitter. She made a scrapbook for us with all of the pictures she took over the year of the kids. My mind has been in a fog, but at least my sense of humor stayed intact for the most part.

I've been amazed at how I've had this village rally around me to support and pray for me. I've also been amazed at the resilience of my children through this and the love and care of my husband and parents. I'm truly blessed beyond what I've ever even understood. To all of you, I thank you. You have sustained me and helped me to carry on when I thought I couldn't. Even the strangers who've come up to me offering me hope have been amazing (at times a little creepy, but still amazing).

No one wants to get cancer. I know I certainly didn't. So far, my outcomes are good and things are looking good. I know that some others are not so lucky. Cancer has taught me that there are so many things in life that are incidental and not monumental. If the house is messy, so what? If I don't get that parking space, life won't end. If a bill is paid late, the world doesn't come raining down. People have arguments, but there is forgiveness. I've learned not to worry about what other people think. I've learned that taking life one day at a time is really all you can do sometimes. I can't worry about tomorrow or what wrongs I have done in the past. It's not worth it. All I can do is live for today. Plan for tomorrow, but live for today. Life can change in a moment.

One of my favorite poems by Jenny Joseph, "When I'm an Old Woman I Shall Wear Purple."

WHEN I'M AN OLD WOMAN I SHALL WEAR PURPLE
With a red hat which doesn't go, and doesn't suit me.
And I shall spend my pension on brandy and summer gloves
And satin sandals, and say we've no money for butter.
I shall sit down on the pavement when I'm tired
And gobble up samples in shops and press alarm bells
And run my stick along the public railings
And make up for the sobriety of my youth.
I shall go out in my slippers in the rain
And pick the flowers in other people's gardens
And learn to spit

You can wear terrible shirts and grow more fat
And eat three pounds of sausages at a go
Or only bread and pickle for a week
And hoard pens and pencils and beermats and things in boxes

But now we must have clothes that keep us dry
And pay our rent and not swear in the street
And set a good example for the children.
We must have friends to dinner and read the papers.

But maybe I ought to practice a little now?
So people who know me are not too shocked and surprised
When suddenly I'm old, and start to wear purple.

■

I think we finally have a fresh start out to the New Year. I feel rested and relaxed after the excitement on New Year's Eve. I spent most of the day on Saturday recovering. My body still aches and it takes a while to get going. But I'm starting to do my yoga-like stretches again like I used to. I used to be able to not only touch my toes, but put my whole palm on the floor. I tried that last night, but it didn't quite work.

Last night while I watched my daughter closely in the bathtub in our bathroom, I started to play around with the wig I'd bought before I lost my hair. The new wig I have on order looks a little more like my natural hair and length before it fell out. I went to wigs.com and they even had videos on how to wear them. The one that's coming in the mail is supposed to be able to be curled, straightened, and all that stuff. I put the wig I have on—which by the way was about $480.00, compared to the one I just ordered for $160—and started to play with it. It kind of flips out on the sides, so I thought I could curl it a bit. So, for the first time in months I took out my curling iron and plugged it in.

I did the first curl on the side and immediately I hear a hissing sound. AAHHHH. I just singed the hair on my wig that I haven't even worn but once. I tried to comb it out and then trim it up. It looks like total bed head in one spot. After this, I took out the instructions that came with the wig. "Do not use any curling or straightening irons on the wig. Do not comb while wet." Well, of course when I singed it, I thought if I wet it, it would help. Yeah. It didn't. Nevertheless, I was able to style it to my liking and even do a little up do with a hair clip. I have to say that I look completely like my mother with it on. Not that it's a bad thing.

Putting on fake eyelashes is a bit tricky. This time I read the directions, so at least I wouldn't use superglue or something like that. You have to somehow put adhesive on the lashes—a very thin layer—and then press them on to your eyelid. This is a lot trickier than it sounds. It's also a little creepy. It's like putting little spiders on your face. Once I got them on, they stayed amazingly and didn't look too bad. I put my wig on in the "up do" position and I have to say, I didn't look as much like a drag queen as I expected.

Of course, my husband and everyone else in the house thought I looked weird because they're used to seeing me with no hair, and for the past while, no eyelashes. By the time I got home, my one eyelash felt like it was coming off. I immediately took off the wig and eyelashes.

I ventured out and no one seemed to stare at me like, "Oh my! That woman has fake hair and eyelashes!" The other great thing is that, because it's unseasonably cold right now, I didn't have a hot flash and the wig actually kept my head warm!

I'm a bit sore and wore out from my outing, but it's a start. I heard from someone that their mother had to take a nap every day for about a year after chemo. I can see that. Naps are good. And they will be much better when I don't have boulders for a chest. I'm totally looking forward to my last major surgery on Friday, January 21st. It will be a day outpatient surgery where they switch out the expanders for the implants.

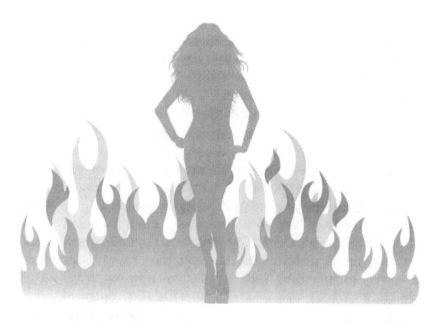

40 IMPLANTS & A VISIBLE END
January 5-25, 2011

On Thursday, before lunch with a girlfriend, I actually decided to do a "mall walk", so I walked the whole entire mall. It took about an hour, but I was right there with the "mature" crowd. I was really surprised to see how many people were out mall walking. Of course, in the afternoon I had to go lay down, but that is progress.

I also got the new wig in the mail. It came out a little darker than I expected, but is about the length of my hair before I lost it all. I tried it on and it didn't look too bad. It even has darker roots to really make it look real. Now I have two wigs for various occasions. How exciting.

Today, I had to leave the house to meet with someone related to my business, so I put on my older wig and false eyelashes! I had to first drop off my daughter at her therapy center. When the therapists saw me walking by, they didn't recognize me! Leaving the house also meant that I had to put on something other than yoga pants. Guess what? My skinny jeans I got last year for Christmas actually fit! I don't even think they fit when I bought them!

After my meeting, I actually went out to lunch with my husband...by ourselves! We haven't done that in ages. It was quite nice. I did take off the wig for the event and went back to the ball cap. I'm still not used to the wig wearing, and I don't think my husband is, either. The new one I got is really big hair, so I'll have to play around with that one for a while.

■

I'm scheduled to get my implants at the end of the week! I'm really hoping that my husband doesn't pay off the surgeon to put in double D's. That would be bad.

My hair is growing back in. I think it might be my original color before I messed with it with highlighting and coloring it, strawberry blonde. Also, my eyelashes are coming back, so I think the products I bought to help with hair and eyelash growth might actually be working. I haven't felt the need to wear the fake eyelashes.

I'm afraid with surgery at the end of the week, I'll lose the energy I've had over the past couple of days. Surgery tends to do that. However, I'm told that this surgery should be pretty easy, especially since I'm in mild pain most of the time with expanders now. Of course, Nurse Hatchet aka my mother, comes back in on Tuesday, but since I'm feeling so good, we're hoping to do some things like have a lunch where I don't feel like I have to lie down afterward. Maybe I'll actually get to enjoy myself a little bit, or rather, my mother will get to enjoy her visit instead of having to be the nurse the whole time.

■

I had my surgery. Whoever told me that it wasn't going to hurt was very wrong. Apparently, the surgeon had to do some fancy handiwork to make sure I was even by manipulating the pocket where the implant goes. That part hurt. In addition, my anesthesiologist was not my favorite. He didn't give me the happy shot until I was on the operating room table and I woke up shivering horribly. I even had to use my old breathing techniques to get my body under control it was so bad.

The night of surgery I was throwing up really bad, had a headache, and couldn't urinate. Obviously, the anesthesiologist didn't do his job. Not even the pain medication touched my headache, and I haven't thrown up like that even during chemotherapy. I got no sleep. I pretty much don't remember Saturday as I was drugged up and trying to recover from the evening symptoms.

The good news is that the surgery center staff was wonderful, as was my surgeon. I'm still quite swollen, but it feels so much better than having the expanders on my chest. I'm even and he nipped and tucked where needed. I think my husband was a little disappointed that I didn't come out looking like Dolly Parton, which is fine with me. Obviously, if he paid off the surgeon, that was a waste of money. I'm about the same size as I was before the cancer. Of course, when you see me, you'll obviously notice that. A friend of mine who had breast cancer said that usually people look down at her chest when they say hi to her now.

They wrapped me up in big bandages, which I got to take off yesterday. I actually got a nice sports bra out of the deal that doesn't look like something my grandmother would wear, or I should say, something that even my grandmother would wear. Most of the weekend I rested and was in bed, taking my medication as instructed. I decided that after I had the problems with the hysterectomy from doing too much too soon, I would actually rest so I'd recover faster.

I'm hoping to set up an exercise program after the doctor says I'm clear. Apparently, you're not supposed to do a lot after this type of surgery because you don't want to change the symmetry of the breasts.

Once I'm healed up, I plan on hitting the mall and buying myself some new clothes. Since I've been living in yoga pants for a year, this should be quite the adventure. I will also have to be refitted for a bra once the swelling goes down.

Next week, I have my three-month follow-up appointments with the oncologist and the breast surgeon. I'm going to try not to focus on recurrence before then. That seems to be at the back of my mind, especially since this cancer goes to the lungs and the bones. Those are not exactly places that you can feel. You have to be scanned.

I've been doing more work and that makes me feel normal. I get really tired, but I'm taking so many supplements. I'm sure that Whole Foods will soon have a personalized parking spot for me. The other thing is to start focusing on my kids and husband and actually enjoying where I'm living. However, I think that cancer is one of those things that unfortunately is always in the back of your mind. I still have to work through it. If I don't have my wig on, people come up to me and make supportive comments. I'm not ready to be the poster child for breast cancer just yet.

I think I will focus more on being the poster mom for autism for my kids for a while. A nice diversion technique.

41 FOLLOW-UP APPOINTMENTS
January 27 — February 7, 2011

Yesterday, I had my follow-up appointment with Dr. Plastic Surgeon, and apparently, I'm healing up nicely. I was excited about the size I am, but they're swollen and have yet to go down. I still have to wear the secure sports bra to make sure that the new pockets he formed for me will not get out of place. Next up will be nipple creation, but not for about six to eight weeks. He can also do some nip and tucks in the office. How's that for health care? Maybe I can get some free Botox while I'm at it.

Now any news, clothing, or medication, the sound of a medical office, facing this thing without a face, has got me on edge. Anything that has to do with cancer, I see as relative to me. Perhaps before I was diagnosed, I didn't pay as much attention. But this week, for example, the headline on CNN.com seemed more than coincidental. The week after I get the implants and I read about how women who get silicone implants have a higher chance of some type of lymphoma. Six days out from getting silicone implants, and someone in a newsroom announces my new risks.

Instead of freaking out and going on Medline and reading every article there is on this topic, I decided to bring the article in to discuss with Dr. Plastic Surgeon. He assured me that my silicone implants are not the same and that he already talked to some "Well-known people in this area," and told me that I shouldn't be worried. I told him the only reason why I worry is that the type of cancer I had—if it's going to spread—it'll spread to the lungs and bones—not exactly an easy place to detect cancer unless you get regular screenings. The same was true of lymphoma.

In my first bold step in not letting the fear of recurrence of cancer rule my life, I threw out the copies I had made of the article before I left the doctor's office.

I'm seeing the beginnings of life going on after cancer. I was outside in the morning, and after the kids got on the bus, some neighbors stopped to chat. I'd met them before the cancer, but it was nice to actually talk to someone and not feel like I had to run inside to pass out. I ate at a new restaurant this week. I wore my wig out. There are moments when I'm still in disbelief that this whole cancer thing has even happened to me and how sick I've been the last year. It feels like a dream, really. But you know what? Life goes on. I'm sure there is a reason for this whole thing that I won't get for a long time.

■

I went to my three-month follow-up appointment with my breast surgeon yesterday. Remember this is the surgeon that I originally went to, and she's wonderful. She got the whole "team" together to get what I feel is the best care possible. Let me back up: If you recall I just had surgery to put my implants in about 10 days ago. On Saturday, I overdid it and did a bunch of work that I probably shouldn't have. Before I went to the appointment, I was completely exhausted. I had a three-hour nap before I even went. Obviously, I was exhausted and not my usually perky self before I went.

Once at Dr. Breast Cancer Surgeon's office, everything was good. I was joking with the MA and put on my silk purple cape so that Dr. Breast Cancer Surgeon could exam me in my superhero form. When she entered in the room and looked at my chest, she looked a little perplexed because I'm still swollen and bruised from the implant surgery. She told me that she thought "We would be farther along than this." I reminded her that I had the infected expander and it had to be put back in, which added several weeks to recovery before the implants could go back in.

She started to examine me around the area of the implants and pointed out a place on my left breast (the cancer side) that there is a tiny spot—that might even be a mole under the skin. At this point, I have so much scar tissue going on in that spot that it really is hard to feel. I mean, after all, I've been under the knife at least five or more times in the last year. She goes on to tell me that I'm in menopause because of my complete hysterectomy. The fatigue is a big part of it in the beginning. She was trying to be nice, but I want to hear when I'll be the energizer bunny again—not that I'm going to have to slow down like I'm 80 years old.

My next appointment with her will be in three months, and she said that hopefully by then she can really get a baseline. Well, the ride home from that appointment sucks. Of course, my mind goes everywhere from "Why doesn't she just take it out now?" to "I can't go through what I just went through the last year again!"

By the time I got home, I was an emotional time bomb. Of course, the first person I see is my babysitter and I burst into tears on her. Poor thing, but she's been with us for a year and a half so far, so she's used to it. My mom gets on the phone and says what I know intellectually: If there was something there it would have shown up on the PET scan. I know that I'm still swollen from the surgery. I know that I overdid it and am exhausted. My mom reiterates that my aunt and anyone else who has cancer goes through this post-treatment emotional rollercoaster.

Here I am in the home stretch and one phrase from a doctor can throw me off. It's the damn terminology on paper versus what I feel inside. I forgot that once you have cancer many people have the breakdown after the fact because you have to have your game face on for all of the treatment, surgeries, and appointments. There is no time really to think about what you're actually going through. Once again, cancer sucks no matter how you slice it.

You have to stay tough during the treatments and then you fall apart looking back at what actually happened to you. Of course, being Superwoman and super adorable, I thought for sure I would be immune to such fallbacks. Apparently not. Becoming a cancer patient is human, going through it's human, and being able to step back and say, *I've been there* is a blessing. There are still so many things that remind me that I'm still "a cancer patient" for a while longer—like the fatigue, having a cold hang on longer, my nails look horrible, and of course my hair—not to mention I still have huge incisions healing on my breasts.

I'm counting my blessings.

■

I saw a commercial for the three-day walk for breast cancer this morning. I still don't think I'm ready to wave that pink flag yet. I'm still too close to it. It's like when my kids were diagnosed with autism. It took a while before I got comfortable with the idea. I think, somewhere in the back of my mind, that if I just get on the pink train that my focus will be on cancer and I'm more apt for recurrence. I know that sounds crazy. I think when my hair grows back more and all of the surgeries are done, I'll feel better about it. We're coming up on a year now that I'll have been dealing with this, and that boggles my mind.

This past week I actually started back to work with my wig in tow. It was great seeing patients again, but exhausting at the same time. The good news is that I didn't have to take a nap. The bad news is I have a lot of work to catch up on. Although I was seeing patients, I used to do a million things at once, making phone calls and writing reports in-between each patient. However, I've been trying to scale back so I don't get so exhausted and ease myself into face time with actually therapy and assessment patients. People are still as crazy as ever and, thus, I'm still in business. I spoke to one patient this weekend whose father is a grave digger. She laughed and said, "He'll never run out of business." Same thing with psychology.

It was wonderful to see a lot of my friends in the field. They loved my wig. As usual, things had not changed much around the place where I perform autism assessments. It really makes you think about how time goes by. Things are still the same at that place. Another indication how important it's to make time in your life for the moment and step out of the day-to-day routine of things. Otherwise, life just ticks away.

I have an appointment with the plastic surgeon this week and then the big follow-up with my oncologist the next week. I haven't decided if I'll wear the wig then or not. I generally just wear it when I'm seeing patients. My hair is coming out spiky-looking. In a month, I might even be able to ditch the wig.

■

I had a follow-up appointment with my plastic surgeon today. I told him about the drama I had after the breast surgeon appointment. He said that he never saw anything in the chart that something was "being watched." I told him that I was just not going to worry about it. He didn't feel anything, and thought that maybe what she was feeling was scar tissue from the expander. He said that he didn't feel anything suspicious or obviously he would have done something about it— particularly since I'm the adorable and favorite patient.

I had to start paying my deductible for the start of the year. I had already paid some of it to the plastic surgeon and the hospital in anticipation of the charges. When I went in to pay my last amount for the surgeon, they wrote it off. How great is that?

I don't have another appointment with him until April. He said that we have to make sure that my implants have "settled" before we do the nipple reconstruction or else I might have nipples that point to the sky. That would be interesting. He called it "skin origami." I think it must be something that plastic surgeons get very excited about, probably how a psychologist feels when they get a new diagnostic case similar to the ones on *House*.

■

This week, I had the three-month follow-up with my oncologist. This means I have to enter the cancer den again where I'd had all of those treatments, which was strange. This time it wasn't so bad walking into the place, and it wasn't that crowded. Sitting in the office and waiting for the doctor, I couldn't believe I was there again. It all seems like a blur.

There were different people at the desk than usual. I was sure the place was going to have that smell I became used to, but I couldn't smell anything. When the medical assistant brought me back, she was a familiar face. Everyone else was the same, including the guy who draws the blood, and the nurses. It was nice. They all remembered me and commented on how my hair was growing back. I had to get on the scale. I gained six pounds since my lowest chemo diet weight, which really isn't that bad.

Dr. Perky and her sidekick, the physician's assistant, came in and gave me hugs. She examined me and said that everything looked great. Since I was having a cold, she didn't want to take the tumor markers because even a cold can elevate the numbers.

Dr. Perky wants me to start taking an aspirin every day though—like the old people in the commercials! Apparently research is saying that it can reduce your likelihood of any type of cancer. It was also requested that I get a bone scan in July to see what damage chemo has done to my bones. Since I live on that island of denial, I forget what my body has been through. She said that it can take over a year for the cells to recover from the event called cancer. She then basically said that was it and to come back in three more months. What? That's it? After being monitored so closely for so long, it's hard to believe that I'm only supposed to go back in three months. She told me to go out and enjoy my life.

She also told me a story about a group of patients that she had several years ago—about five patients, all of whom had breast cancer and chemotherapy. Several months after they completed chemotherapy, all five of their husbands dropped dead. She said that the women were more depressed over that then the breast cancer. Her moral of the story was to go out and enjoy life right now, because you don't know what the future holds. How's that for a pep talk? Even the PA was looking at her like, "What're you talking about?"

As I left the Cancer Center, it dawned on me why Dr. Perky is so perky. She really does take her own advice and live each day to the fullest. Instead of letting the work she does get her down, she allows it to revitalize her life. She lives each day to the fullest and does not let anything get her down because she realizes that any day could be her last. It was like a lightbulb went off in my head. (Well, a dim one, since I still have a head cold.) What a freeing thought.

Let today take care of today and let tomorrow take care of itself. I knew that, but it sank in a little bit more after that appointment. The energy that I've wasted in my life worrying about what would happen tomorrow could fuel a jet plane; it's not worth it. Yes, my cancer might come back. Yes, I might be hit by a truck tomorrow, but, I can't spend my time worrying about that. If I have to deal with that in the future then I will worry about it then. God only gives us the grace we need to handle what we need to for today.

Later, I walked into the salon at Ulta and decided to get my hair done. I haven't had it done in over a year now. I told the girl that I didn't want to look like an old lady with stripped hair and I want to grow it out. I ended up with a head full of foils. When she took them out, I told her I look like I have a girlfriend named "Madge." She laughed. Everyone in the salon was saying how adorable it looked. She styled it into a pixie cut. I'm convinced that when I went to the bathroom, she paid everyone to say that.

I got home and looked at myself in the mirror and didn't know who it was. I decided that maybe more makeup might make me look like Michelle Williams. But it was not Michelle Williams in the mirror, and it definitely was not me. I guess trying to recognize who you're after all of this is exactly what they mean by moving on.

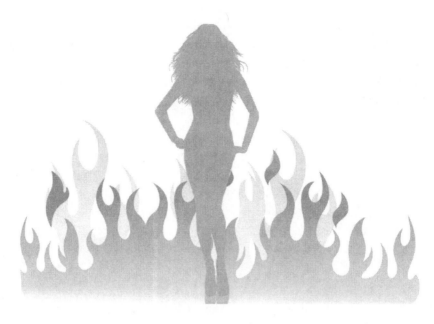

42 COUNTDOWN TO 1-YEAR
ANNIVERSARY

March — April 2011

My energy is definitely coming back. I'm not winded running up the stairs. It has been weeks since I felt dizzy from just getting up. I can actually taste the wonderful blessing of food. The ridges in my nails from chemo are just about all grown out, and the horizon of a pedicure is near. I don't need a nap every day. But all it takes to remind me of my ordeal is one look in the mirror. My battle scars and my hair growth are reminders of the last year. The hot flashes and insomnia are déjà vu of difficult days passed.

The mirror has come to depict me in the way that cancer sees fit. While I remain myself on the inside, my eyes struggle to reach consensus with my reflection. As a result, my inner conscious is brewing up a fight to reclaim my image. This week, I actually saw some patients without my wig. I'm getting tired of it because it's getting warmer. I was really nervous about walking into the office without it, but everyone said that I have enough hair that it looks good—even "edgy", as one person said.

I really find myself not wanting to look back at the past year, nor be reflective. I thought that I would be more in a "what I've learned from cancer" mode. I definitely think there are several things that I've learned, but the desire to return to some type of normalcy is more of a goal at this point.

The medical assistant who checked me in for my last oncology appointment is also dealing with breast cancer. Of course, she works at a cancer center, but she was decked out in all of the ribbons and bracelets that said, "I love boobs! Save the boobs." I'm still not ready to make that kind of statement, to be a public warrior. I'm still searching for peace within me, reorganizing myself to return to a normal life of being a psychologist, mother, wife, and daughter. I need to find the light within me before I go and shine brightly; I have to shine for me first. But I've found that if I'm too reflective about the year (it's hard for me to say about the cancer), then I start second-guessing myself. For example, did I really need all of the chemo? A lot of people just have a bilateral mastectomy and don't do the chemo. I don't think I could have done just a lumpectomy because I would then be wondering if it would return in the other breast. Was I really as sick as I was?

I know I was, and I know I did the right thing and made all of the right decisions in terms of my care. But the question of *what if* is always lurking. What if I never got it checked out in the first place? If I think too hard about the series of events, the doubts start to cast their gray where there should be light. It's not so much as taking things for granted, it's just how precarious being a cancer victim can be. I've gone from sometimes having my medical status literally checked hourly to only once every three months. It's really a difficult transition mentally when on paper it could happen instantly.

∎

It's April, which means this month marks a year ago that I started the process that led to my diagnosis. I tell patients all the time that when the anniversary of a traumatic event comes up, we naturally get depressed or sad. I don't know that I'm depressed, but I'm definitely in disbelief. May 4th is just around the corner. I've been feeling really good, so I think that helps. There are the lingering signs of what I've been through that can't be denied. The most obvious is my hair. Every time I go past a window or a mirror, I wonder who that passing shadow is.

I have the scar where my port was placed that can be seen most of the time. Then there are the other surgical scars that are under my clothes. Of course, there are my new implants and my complete lack of feeling in the breast area. The hot flashes are also a constant reminder. One of the nice things about being on all of the happy drugs that come along with chemo meant that I could sleep or take a nap on a moment's notice.

My sleep pattern is completely disrupted. Taking naps is hard, and I can't fall asleep without my happy pill. I hope that I have not become dependent on these little pills as a source of rest. And emotionally, I don't know if the full impact of what has happened to me has set in. Maybe it never will. I was never a person to linger on the past, even though its marks lingered on my body.

This week I received a magazine called *Cure*, that's for cancer patients, survivors, and caretakers. It's an excellent magazine that has a summary of a lot of the research that's out there. This month's headline was "Chemobrain." I know I've mentioned chemo brain in the past, but it was nice to see that it's real. I still have some it going on.

My body does not recover as quickly as it did before I got sick. Things linger. Hangovers used to last a couple of hours. Now it takes a good day if not more. Not to mention my short-term memory is completely shot.

One of my aunts was recently re-diagnosed with breast cancer. I wonder what her thoughts were when she was counting down to her own anniversary? Was cancer counting down its return simultaneously? This scares me more than anything.

I remember thinking when I was sick—like most of us probably would—that when I got better, I would totally start taking better care of myself. I planned in my mind that I would be working out, eating healthy, and would completely overhaul my life. Well, I think since I've been better, chocolate, wine, frosting, donuts, and tasty, fattening meals have won out! One reason, of course, is that I haven't been able to have any of that for a long time. My stomach is still a little sensitive, but I've pushed through it. A friend of mine has been talking to me about seeing her doctor who specializes in natural remedies, chelation, and the like to maximize health. Will this prevent cancer from coming back? I don't know. But I know with my kids' problems, I have literally tried everything in hopes of helping them. Why not give the same energy to myself? After all, I do hope to be around for a very long time.

I guess I'm a cancer survivor. I haven't mentally put myself in that category yet. After all, when exactly does that start? My aunt was a survivor. Now she's gone back to being a patient. That's the problem with the terminology, they don't fit all body types or cancer types. Did I become a survivor after I had the mastectomy or after my chemo stopped? It's hard to tell, but in the end, it's me who will make it official. I was reading in the magazine that some people just "live" with cancer. I should be lucky that I only needed six rounds of chemo—not 12 or more like some people.

∎

Today, I had a follow-up appointment with my plastic surgeon. I'm slated to get new and exciting nipples. I don't know how exciting that's going to be since, again, I'm completely numb in that area. I went to the office and was greeted with my usual good spirits of adorableness by the staff. They commented about how long it had been since they saw me. It does feel kind of long.

Once I was in the room, I put on the gown once again. It gave me flashbacks of all of the times I was in the hospital. In the exam room, there's a large floor to ceiling mirror. As I undressed, I was able to get a full view of my new chest. GASP! To my surprise, my right breast looks larger and lower than my left! Ugh. I didn't notice this before! I usually get dressed in the closet and, with small children running around, I don't walk around naked in front of the mirrors at home.

Once the surgeon came in, I pointed this out, and he actually started to go through the chart to see if he put in different sizes! He backpedaled, saying that it's only been three months since the surgery and it takes about that time or longer for the swelling to go down, so maybe that is what's going on. Obviously lopsided boobs is not as bad as having cancer. I can certainly live with it. At least they're perky. But still, this feels like something else I have to deal with when I'm desperately trying to live in denial of the last 12 months. My shoulder and chest muscles ache if I don't sit up straight. It's the strangest sensation to lift something up and have mysterious mounds retract when your muscles move.

After I went to the surgeon's office, I went over to my oncologist's office to get my blood drawn for my tumor levels. I walked into the office and, as I did, a woman who was bald wearing a baseball cap passed me by. That was me months ago. How I remember those days—practically living in the office with chemo. Again, it hasn't been that long—only six months—since my last chemo. Can you believe it? I only had one vial of blood drawn. I almost felt cheated. It's a strange feeling to have every bodily function monitored daily and then go to only seeing your "team" every few months. They send you on your way telling you to live your life. And out the door I go, trying to make sense of it all. Easier said than done.

■

My oncologist's office called to let me know that my tumor markers were normal! This is great news. These last two weeks of April mark the anniversary of my medical work-up before my diagnosis. I can clearly remember standing in the shower, doing my own breast exam and feeling the lump. I hate to think if I would have procrastinated on getting medical treatment or a mammogram. These days when I'm in the shower and continue to do breast exams, it's more difficult trying to figure out what's what since I have the implants.

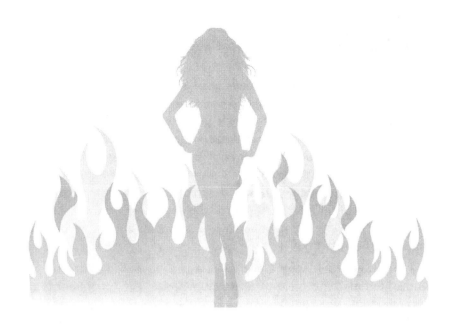

43 MOVING ON

May 2011

This week marks a year ago that I was diagnosed with cancer. My hair is growing longer thanks to "Ovation Cell Therapy" shampoo. I'm getting stronger each day.

I was invited by a new friend to attend the Relay for Life event sponsored by the American Cancer Society this weekend. She said that I would be one of the honored survivors and that she'd introduce me to some people. I agreed to go, but when I glanced at the website, I realized that this would be a new step in my journey against cancer. It was time to move on, and more difficult than moving on, to do so publicly.

When I registered, they gave me a purple "survivor" t-shirt and a purple wristband. There were several other people with the purple shirt, most of them older women. I was relieved when I saw a woman I know who's also a survivor. During the opening ceremonies, they had all of the purple shirts come up and get a medal, then a local radio personality spoke about surviving prostate cancer. There was hardly a dry eye in the place. Then, all the survivors had to make a lap around the park area to celebrate our "victory" lap. I have to say, I thought I was going to lose it. There were people of all ages, but it looked like I was the only one with short hair that was not cut and styled. I was one of the few newly-recovering people.

One of the women said she had cancer four years ago. I immediately asked her more about her hair because it was so long. Next was a special dinner for just the survivors. I got to meet a lot of other women who battled breast cancer several years ago. One woman told me she had intensive radiation for 10 days; it took her almost three years to recover from the fatigue. When I mentioned forgetting things and having to write stuff down, they all laughed and said that they definitely still have a lot of that. It was comforting in a way, but a club that I really wish I didn't belong to; membership was forced, but this dinner was completely voluntary.

Around the track, where everyone would be walking into the wee hours of the morning, were dedicated luminaries. The "in honor of" and "in memory of" on the bags were a little depressing. The glow of those words revealed the power of what I had faced, my adversary who had certainly waged a war on not only my body, but had claimed others not as fortunate as I was. It was an eerie reality that was absent from the spa-designed doctor's offices or the perky attending nurses. This track depicted the solitary journey I had in my mind, upon which my thoughts raced and raced as the journey neared completion.

Denial is a part of surviving sometimes. Seeing the track and meeting survivors helped build a sense of solidarity. After dinner, I walked back over to my friend and tried to forget that I was wearing a purple shirt. Another woman came up with a purple shirt and started to tell me her experiences. It was nice, but still a lot more emotional than I thought it would be. I didn't stay much longer after that. I guess in some ways, my denial is not as strong as I thought it was.

I'm glad I went, as emotional as it was. It taught me that a lot of people several years out from cancer are doing great. I learned that I have something to look forward to and that the journey is not necessarily just a dark one. I heard one woman say that cancer was a blessing. I don't think I'm at that point, but I can see what she means. I've learned over the past several months to slow down and quit working when I'm tired. I've learned not to worry so much about stuff. If you don't have your health, the little stuff in life becomes rough. If the house is messy, oh well. If I don't get done everything I needed to do today, it'll still be there tomorrow. I don't have to see everyone who calls and needs a psychologist. I'm learning to work smarter, not harder. I can take a day off, and the world won't end. Things don't have to be perfectly organized. Not everyone has to see things my way. Cancer teaches you a lot.

This weekend helped me to see that talking about cancer doesn't kill me.

■

On Monday, I had a follow-up appointment with my breast surgeon. It was pretty uneventful—which is good. She actually wanted me to wait a year to come back. I said, "No way." I told her that I need to come back in six months. I like my safety net.

As I left, one of the girls called me on my phone because she hadn't come out to say hello to me while I was there. She didn't recognize me because I had hair! She was going on about how good I looked and that my hair got long so fast. How sweet was that?

I find myself able to talk more about having cancer the last year with other people, but it's usually related to explaining why my hair is so short. I guess do I have some vanity in me after all.

My next obsession seems to be my skin. Before I got diagnosed I had an appointment to see a dermatologist to make sure I didn't have any pre-cancerous stuff going on. I cancelled it. It just seemed like too much to deal with and to be honest, it still does. However, I should get over there since I'm in the sun more than last year and every freckle I get I'm scrutinizing. Since my PET scan was clear and my tumor markers are back to normal, I'm not too worried. Just the usual hypochondria kind of thing. I guess I should make that appointment again.

I've also actually read a couple of fiction books in the past weeks.

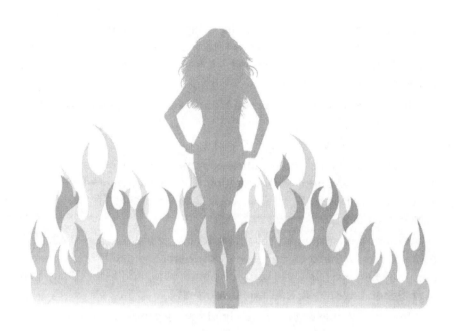

44 LIVING IT UP

June — July 2011

I'm actually trying to live it up this summer since I was in bed and bald all last summer! I've actually been in the pool on an almost daily basis! It's been wonderful. I'm eating my way through lost time now. I don't think that there's a piece of chocolate safe in my presence. Also, don't offer me any cake with frosting. I don't have the strength to turn it down. As a matter of fact, I'm thinking that one of my trips should be to Hoboken, New Jersey, just so I can get a fondant cake from *Cake Boss*!

I just got back from a trip to Illinois to visit my family. This was the first time in two years. It was wonderful to see them. My mom had a party on Sunday for all the relatives. We were able to go to Chicago, the Lincoln Park Zoo, and Navy Pier. I kept thinking the whole time that I would never have made it past the parking lot last year since I was so weak. I was able to walk for literally what seemed like miles. I made sure that I ate all of the Chicago delights, like Lou Malnetti's Pizza and Italian beef.

This month, I have to follow up with bloodwork and get their requested bone scan to see what damage chemo has done.

I still get *Cure* magazine for patients, caretakers, and professionals in the cancer field. Last time I got it, I didn't want to read it. I don't like to think about being a cancer survivor, but this month I did. There was a lot of interesting stuff, and I also had the concentration to actually read a whole article. I did read in one of the local newspapers about a little girl who recently died from a blood-related cancer. Apparently as an infant, she had chemo due to a brain tumor. One of the risks of chemotherapy is that it can cause other cancers. She ended up getting several different types of cancers and then died. Stuff like that will linger in my mind for a while after I read it.

After all, there are so many different types you can get that you don't feel any symptoms until it's too late. I try not to think about that, even though there are lingering thoughts about the realm of this dangerous disease. Instead I really try to focus on the surgeries I had, and if the chemotherapy did their job. My only job is to live life now, for myself, for my husband, for my kids. And even for those whom I work with. Another survivor, after all, is another beam of hope. Studies indicate that a positive attitude is half the battle, right?

Now that summer is almost over, I have my meetings with my oncologist and plastic surgeon. My plastic surgeon will hopefully make me look like a Playboy model—or just not a nipple-less female would be nice. My oncologist's office was supposed to call me to set up a blood draw and a bone scan, but they haven't yet. I will have to call them myself, which is odd. I go from daily phone calls from that office to being neglected. I guess that's one area for which I'm glad I'm not the priority anymore!

My kids go back to school tomorrow, and I got to go to the "Meet the Teacher" event on Friday.

This summer was great despite its challenges. I guess when you're not in bed all day, you have to interact with the world. And there, it's more likely you'll face obstacles. But these past few months, I really tried to get out more and hang out with my kids and husband.

And guess what?

We went to Disneyland.

■

I was reading an article in the paper this week called "My So-called Midlife." The gist is it's about a 40-something year old woman talking about being 40-something. When I first started reading it, I assumed it was about an old lady until it dawned on me that, in a couple of weeks, I, too, will be 40-something. Ain't that a bitch?

She discussed the grueling task of finding a pair of jeans that fit. In her discussion, she noted how her body has significantly changed over the past several years. Ugh! This is something that I seem to be facing. My chemo diet is long gone, but the lost pounds are back. Somehow, my clothes seem to fit differently than before chemo. Not only did my body survive cancer, but it also survived two children. If back fat is part of that deal, so be it.

I'm ready for the final reconstruction portion of my surgeries. I met with my plastic surgeon and I have healed enough that we can proceed with the nipples. The plastic surgeon is quite excited as he will get to do his "skin origami", as you see, nipple making is an art form. The folds, the sculpting, and that "aha" moment when the artist steps back to admire a new creation is his delight. The last several times I've seen my surgeon who keeps asking, "Did I put different sizes in?" I have to remind him that he didn't. Apparently on the left side where the cancer was, they were more aggressive with taking out tissue. The right side where the expander was infected probably has more tissue and more scar tissue as well, making it look larger. Much to my husband's delight, the surgeon wants to change out the smaller implant for a bigger one. So, this will be yet another day at the surgery center. I'm not really worried about the pain or anything like the last surgeries; my breasts are pretty much numb. If I get too close to the stove without noticing, I would probably burn myself. I don't imagine the recovery is going to be too bad.

In the midst of planning for my next surgery, I finally made it to the dermatologist for a "body mapping." I'm very fair-skinned—in some lights, actually blue. I also went because over the past couple of weeks, I developed a weird pink thing on my chest. It was weirdly shaped and raised. Just what I needed to worry about—skin cancer. I was very good and didn't let my mind go there, but still, given that I found my breast cancer on my own, I wasn't waiting for my general practitioner to find this one.

I went to the appointment and, of course, I have to completely undress. At this point, so many people have seen me naked over the past year that I have no shame. The medical assistant that checked me in reminded me that they see all types of bodies and it's no news to them anymore, either. The doctor comes in with her other medical assistant, who's clicking away at the computer. Then the typical small talk starts to happen as my privates are examined, upon which she starts to look more closely at my skin.

She measures my more prominent moles and looks between my toes. I'm glad my feet were manicured. Then I show her the thing on my chest. She starts rattling off some possible things it might be, including basal cell carcinoma, which is the most common form of skins cancer. She didn't really say, "Don't worry, I'm sure that is not it." Before I know it, I'm on the table getting a needle in my skin and the doctor shaves off whatever it is. It was like going to In-N-Out Burger, but a lot quicker.

By the time I get to my imaginary drive-through window, it turns out I didn't have skin cancer. It's just some type of benign keloid. You can bet that I'll be going back to the dermatologist a little more often now.

When I pass by a mirror, I have to admit that I wonder who the heck that woman is staring back at me. Although my hair is longer, it's still not long enough to be cut in some cute style yet. I remember when in my pre-surgery fright, I had colored it on my own, had it fixed up by Not-So-Normal Girl, and then it started to fall out. Here I was, still in front of a mirror. I hope that the gel and mousse will create some type of look that seems on purpose. I made it this far, after all.

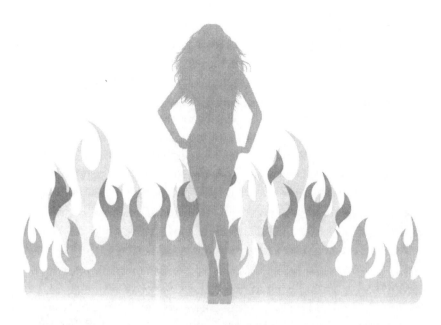

45 BREAST RECONSTRUCTION
September 2011

This week, I had another surgery to reconstruct my breasts into a new type of splendor. The goal was to have a new implant put in on the right side. A couple of my friends have commented on how nonchalant I have been about the surgery. Given that my breasts are pretty much numb, I didn't really think too much about having surgery other than the excitement of having happy drugs in my medicine cabinet again. However, after considering that he was going to replace an implant and nip and tuck some of the imperfection, I did tell him that the nipple reconstruction can wait. After all, I would had to go through all of this and have one nipple facing south and the other one pointing north.

I brought this up to my surgeon as he was playing tic-tac-toe on my chest with his happy purple marker before surgery. I'm glad I mentioned this to him. He looked a little haggard and unshaven. Granted, he has a new baby, so who knows how much sleep he had. I got a little worried when I had to remind him that he was replacing one of the implants to even me out. I did want to mention that he could use me as a practice patient if he wanted to do any tummy tuck or liposuction, but given how tired he looked, I figured I better not ask.

The pre-op nurse who checked me in was very nice. Okay, overly nice. She was sweet in the way that someone who hasn't had 15 surgeries in the last year needs someone to be. Since I have hair now, breast reconstruction must have seemed like an elective surgery to her—until she read my chart and realized that I'd been through the ringer in the last year. So, that set off my lecture from her—in the nicest way, of course—of how my diet should be because I "Will always be a cancer patient" from now on.

Yup, that was my bubble of denial being burst. She went on to spend the next 90 minutes telling me why I should be eating more fruits and vegetables, and even starting to "juice." Is that really a verb?

She went as far as to say that I should be drinking water that is alkaline and buying everything organic. She even printed off information for me to reference. I can really see the benefit in theory. She then mentioned that my kids should be eating like that as well. I restrained from mentioning that I'm lucky to get my kids to eat anything since they have autism.

■

So far, my surgery looks like it went well. I'm not in any kind of pain—not that I'm forgoing the pain pills; I'm rather numb. I look pretty even, but who knows until the swelling goes down. I figure if I get enough plastic surgery from the guy, I'm bound to get a tummy tuck for free just so he can practice. Keep your fingers crossed.

I think I can hold off *Playboy* magazine for my cover shoot for at least another couple of months. Besides, since my last experience with my expander getting infected, I'm all about taking things slowly. I have my follow-up appointment with Dr. Plastic Surgeon today and an appointment with my oncologist on Tuesday.

I'll get a bone scan to "see what chemo has done to my bones" and a general follow-up. I personally think that she could have put that in perkier terms like "We'd like to see how strong your bones are." Something like that.

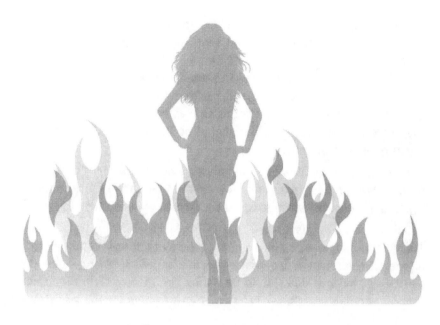

46 THREE YEARS SINCE

September 2013

It's been almost three years since I ended my chemotherapy. My follow-up with my breast surgeon and my oncologist last month went well. My oncologist said that I will see him again in February for possibly my last scan for a while. Of course, that terrifies me because I will be insisting that I continue to have scans! I recently had a patient whose mother had a backache in 2011, and it turned out to be cancer. She was dead within three weeks. I had to probe her about what symptoms she had prior to the backache.

Over the past several months, I've been lamenting the loss of my pre-cancer body and energy level. Although I remain my perky self, I find that I can't sustain the perkiness like I used to. Some tell me that it's actually a function of age, but I'm not so sure. No one talks much about the post-cancer treatment lifestyle. Usually, all of the focus is on the fact that the cancer is gone. This is obviously a fabulous fact, but some days, looking in the mirror at a body that's prematurely aged a decade is not fun to discuss.

My hair isn't growing in as fast as I'd like. I'm not one of the survivors who lucked out to have thick, curly hair come back (I wish!); instead it's finer than it was before. My chemo weight loss plan backfired on me, and I've put on weight. And yes, I now believe that it's harder to lose weight after chemo-induced menopause and a hysterectomy. I apologize to all of those women who I rolled my eyes at when they suggested it was harder to lose and maintain weight after surgery. I'm now on your bandwagon, another reason to "never say never." At times, I feel like I should get a t-shirt that says "I used to be cute, skinny, and have fabulous hair before cancer!" or "I'm not really a soccer mom. I just had chemo."

Funny thing is, when I think back to BC (Before Cancer) I complained about my weight, my hair, and my general appearance at times.

When I meet with my breast surgeon, who's already been through menopause, and discuss my gripes about fatigue, hot flashes, poor muscle tone, and fat in places I didn't know I had fat, she doesn't even give me a pep talk or rally to my side with a magic pill. She just sighs and starts to chime in about how sex and vaginal dryness is no picnic, either. I will spare you the details of this conversation, as I'm hoping that my past chemo-fog erases that one from my memory as well. Instead of hope, she suggested a bone density scan. Great. Not the news I was hoping for. Happy 43rd birthday to me. Damn, that sounds old!

Despite my woes, I remember and remind myself to rejoice that these are wonderful complaints to have instead of the alternative.—not being here. My lovely husband reminds me when I can't fit into my pants and I'm ready to light fire to my closet, that my body has been through an amazing trauma, and I can't expect so much of myself. I'm further reminded that not being able to fit in my BC jeans really is a minor issue by the news that a close family friend, whom I called "aunt" for my entire life, died this week from the cancer that overtook her body in a very short period of time.

So I'm grateful for my post cancer body that keeps me out of the competition of "the best of the soccer moms" and worrying about if I'm a size 6 or not. I'm thankful for my short hair that makes getting ready in the morning a breeze. I'm thankful for my fatigue that reminds me I'm not superwoman and need to slow down and enjoy life more. I'm thankful that I can see the upside of being a cancer survivor. I'm thankful that I'm here to watch by children grow up.

As one of my friends put it over the summer when we were hanging out at the pool, "My kid doesn't care if I'm 100 pounds in a string bikini or 200 pounds in a burka. She only cares that I'm here." It certainly puts things into perspective.

47 FIVE YEARS OUT

May 2015

In May 2015, I made it to the magical five-year mark. Apparently this is the point when I can breathe easier. I have to say that I am extremely grateful that I made it this far. I have learned a lot about myself. I am stronger than I even imagined that I could be. Some things are the same. My hair still is not anywhere close to where it was before cancer. I am pretty sure that I have spent a small fortune on hair products, vitamins and extensions with not a lot of luck. I have a love and hate relationship with my body. I still haven't gotten back into my pre-cancer state and I don't really think it is going to happen unless I go on "The Biggest Loser." I vacillate between wanting to eat healthy and punishing my body for betraying me. I have all of the books and done all of the research on the benefits of a "whole food" diet. I've even cooked a couple of successful "vegan" meals. However, I find it hard to have more than one in a row. I usually return to my chocolate and wine soon thereafter. I have also scoured the Internet to find articles that state "drinking wine fend off cancer." I have yet to find any reliable research on the subject.

My scars are still here. I doubt they are going away anytime soon either. Some days they are a reminder of my strength. On other days, I try not to look hoping that 2010 was really just a dream. I have not completely embraced being a survivor. It feels like if I do embrace it, then the cancer can come back. In psychology we call this type of reasoning "magical thinking." I am aware of it but do it anyway. On the other hand, since having cancer, I don't put up with a lot of crap. I was having dinner with a friend of mine whose husband just overcame colon and liver cancer. He has a road map of scars on his abdomen. She asked me if I get agitated after cancer because he certainly does. She relayed a story where he was fed up with one of his clients and lifted up his shirt to show his scars. Yelling that he had cancer and doesn't need to put up with jerks anymore. When she told me that, I had to laugh. I replied that I definitely get fed up with people and have no problem walking away. I have fantasied about pulling up my shirt to tell someone off, but haven't had the nerve to do that yet. I do have several good lines saved in case anyone makes an undesirable comment about me. I keep waiting for someone to mention something about my hair so I can retort, "Oh, the next time I have cancer I will be sure to consult you about whether being alive or having hair should be my priority." Just waiting to use that one.

I continue to be amazed that check-ups take the wind out of me. When I go in to see my oncologist emotionally I feel like I have to prepare for good or bad news. There is no in between. Everything has been good so far but I'm always waiting for the other shoe to drop. I am exhausted at the end of an appointment and usually have to take a nap. On some level it is like reliving the whole illness again.

Due to multiple life circumstances in the past two years, I have had to switch oncologists. The new doctor is not as aggressive as the ones from the past. As a matter of fact, he expressed that my chemo protocol was probably overkill: easy for him to say. As a result, I have found a third oncologist. Changing doctors feels like starting a new relationship all over.

I have a difficult time now even hearing about other people who have cancer. Just this past month, two acquaintances died very quickly after their cancer came back. Of course, I want the details but I don't. It is like a car wreck and I can't look away. What kind of cancer did they have? Where did it come back? What were their symptoms that led to them going back to the doctor? One woman went to the Emergency Room with back pain. Her cancer came back and was all over her body! Nowadays if I get a hangnail I think it's related to cancer. My back hurts, maybe it's cancer?! I can literally drive myself nuts. Then I start Googling: What are the symptoms of lung cancer? What are the symptoms of bone cancer? At some point, I start utilizing my own psychological techniques. I have to talk myself down and remember to enjoy today. Tomorrow will take care of itself. I'm doing what I need to do.

In some ways cancer prepared me for some "other life circumstances" that I have had to deal with in the past couple of years. Remember earlier when I said that my "adoring husband" was by my side? Well, come to find out that infidelity was the *least* of his transgressions. I actually found out via old emails that *the day* of my mastectomy he left the hospital telling my parents he had a stomach ache to go home (yes, in my house) and sleep with one of his assistants. The doting husband was only a façade. Since finding out about his exploits and other circumstances, I am now a single mom raising two kids with autism. I am faced with the dilemma of filling out a dating profile. Do I check the box that I have had a mastectomy and breast cancer or spice up by adding that I did some "remodeling" in the chest area? Awesome. That should be fun. Be sure to look out for my next book... I am pretty sure there has yet to be a screenplay or Lifetime movie of the week that comes close to my reality.

In conclusion, yes, cancer sucks. Big time. It is not something that happens to you and you easily forget it. It stays with you. Sometimes I think about it all the time. On good days, it is just a passing thought. What has stuck with me is that I am more than my illness. It took cancer for me to truly not sweat the small stuff.

ABOUT THE AUTHOR

Dr. Bailey is a licensed clinical psychologist who has been in the field for over 20 years. She received her doctorate from Illinois School of Professional Psychology at Chicago with an emphasis in Health Psychology.

Her vast career has included crisis team work, individual and family therapy, psychological assessments, public speaking, and teaching. She has taught at community colleges, Pepperdine University, and Ryokan College and Arizona State University.

Dr. Bailey has the distinctive qualifications of having been a licensed

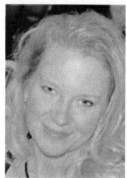

clinical psychologist in hospital, clinic, and private settings, and as a Regional Center consulting psychologist. Her extensive knowledge of available therapies in conjunction with her knowledge of public systems and agencies allows for expert clinical diagnoses, as well as provision of individually-prescribed therapy recommendations. This includes her work as Director of Allied Health for oband Surgery Centers in California, Nevada and Florida.

In addition to her private practice, Dr. Bailey has taken a special interest in the field of autism. She has two children who are on the spectrum, and as a result, she is passionate about helping families with children with special needs.

She is also a breast cancer survivor. Being trained as a health psychologist prepared her with the knowledge to help patients with chronic and terminal issues; her experience as a patient with her own illness gives her a unique perspective to provide unparalleled compassion to her patients.

Visit her website for more information: www.drmelissabailey.com

The Entrepreneur's Publisher

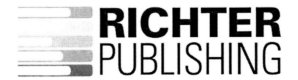

RICHTER
PUBLISHING

CPSIA information can be obtained
at www.ICGtesting.com
Printed in the USA
FFOW02n2308011115
18245FF